S0-BYJ-165

The Smarter Athlete

TO DOCTOR TEBO

MAY YOU BE BLESSED

WITH CONTINUED HEALTH

AND FITNESS

Edmund Burke

The Smarter Athlete

Your Guide to Peak Performance

Eduardo Añorga, MD

iUniverse, Inc.
New York Lincoln Shanghai

The Smarter Athlete
Your Guide to Peak Performance

Copyright © 2006 by Eduardo Añorga

All rights reserved. No part of this book may be used or reproduced by any means, graphic, electronic, or mechanical, including photocopying, recording, taping or by any information storage retrieval system without the written permission of the publisher except in the case of brief quotations embodied in critical articles and reviews.

iUniverse books may be ordered through booksellers or by contacting:

iUniverse
2021 Pine Lake Road, Suite 100
Lincoln, NE 68512
www.iuniverse.com
1-800-Authors (1-800-288-4677)

The information in this book is intended to provide general information about exercise, diet, and training. In addition to offering no guarantees of success or specific results, the information in this book should not be considered to be a substitute for professional assistance with your training program, diet, or medical problems. In certain circumstances exercise and dietary adjustments can be harmful to you health. Before you make any changes in your routine be sure to consult the appropriate professional to confirm that any changes in your routine are recommended for your situation. Likewise, if you have any questions or problems regarding your specific situation it is recommended that you consult the appropriate professional in your area of concern.

ISBN-13: 978-0-595-36435-0 (pbk)
ISBN-13: 978-0-595-80867-0 (ebk)
ISBN-10: 0-595-36435-7 (pbk)
ISBN-10: 0-595-80867-0 (ebk)

Printed in the United States of America

Dedication:

I'd like to extend a special thanks to my family and friends for being so supportive.

Contents

CHAPTER 1

Get in the Right State of Mind

Your mind. We want to talk about it first because it's the most powerful part of your body, and it's where all the decisions are made. Not only is it the control center for all your deliberate actions, your brain also commands the millions of automatic processes that make your life possible. As this highly sophisticated piece of equipment doesn't come with a user's manual, most athletes have had to learn on their own how to develop and maintain an optimal mental state for practice and competition.

Your situation is different. Instead of stumbling through the process on a trial and error basis, you can learn to use a systematic approach to get in the best state of mind to practice and compete.

We can begin by evaluating the choices you make because they will influence your mental state. Decision making is a vital mental function. You either make decisions in a conscious, deliberate manner or you make them automatically, without considering the choices. Many decisions are based on information you gather to evaluate your options. For example, should you drink Diet Coke or 7UP? You make your choice based on what you know about each beverage. You evaluate the factors that you think are important, such as taste, the amount of caffeine, or the amount of sugar. Finally you make a decision.

You make other decisions automatically, without considering the options or even if the options matter. As an example, I am going to ask you to freeze for a moment. That's right. Don't move. Now evaluate how you are currently positioned. What is your posture like right now? How did you end up in that position? Did you know that your posture has a substantial effect on your mood and your level of alertness? When you're trying to learn something new, you can make a choice about how to position yourself. Now, what if good posture could improve your athletic performance by making you feel more alert and confident? You would begin to pay attention to your posture and, with time, that good posture would become a habit. Once we develop a habit, we tend to hold on to it, regardless of whether it is an effective behavior. It takes new information and feedback to draw our attention to an ineffective habit so that we can choose to change our behavior.

To perform at your best, you're going to need good information about training techniques and nutrition, but it doesn't stop there. You will need to know how to develop the habits that keep you confident, motivated, and in the best state of mind to compete.

Sports psychology is the study of how your mind affects your athletic performance. It's a broad subject, and I've decided to focus on five essential areas:

1. Making the choices that will help you build a strong foundation as an athlete
2. Understanding motivation
3. Learning to monitor your thoughts so you can replace negative thoughts with positive thinking
4. Identifying sports-related stress and reviewing strategies for stress management
5. Maintaining the optimal state of mind for practice and competition

Build a Strong Foundation

You're reading this book because you want to learn how to improve your athletic performance. Start with your thoughts, because what you think and believe will ultimately determine your behavior. Your behavior, the way you eat, and how you structure your training program will play a major role in how well you perform.

Your thoughts will follow you into competition and affect your performance both in and out of the arena. Take the home court advantage as an example. Even though most sports have similar playing arenas, the cheering of the crowd and familiarity with the venue will affect how the players perform.

Experienced athletes are able to play at their best even if the crowd is not behind them, but it takes character. Their personal strength and confidence sustains them when the crowd is against them. You can begin to define your character by understanding your thoughts and beliefs because they are what determine how you go about achieving your goals.

Many people believe how they think and act is set in stone. They'll tell you: "That's just the way I am," "I always drop the ball under pressure," or "I always show up late for practice." Even if an approach doesn't work for them, they'll continue using it, because they think that's the way they are. "Never mind that it's harder to hammer a nail in backward. That's the way I do it!"

You have a choice. You can take a step back and look at how your life works. If your approach to a problem isn't working, you can change it. You can change the way you think, and you can change the way you behave.

Being able to change the way you think and behave is good news for athletes who lack confidence in their natural abilities. Although natural talent is valuable, it's definitely not everything. It takes years to master the skill set for a sport, so it will be difficult to know how talented you are until you fully develop your skills. In the long run, the choices you make about how to develop your talents will have the greatest influence on your ability to compete.

What are the choices that will help you build a solid foundation as an athlete? I've grouped them into eight categories:

1. Integrity—the ability to make morally sound decisions
2. Preparedness—developing the foresight to make all the necessary tools available
3. Teamwork—learning how to put the team's goals ahead of individual goals
4. Adaptability—how to keep your composure when things don't go your way
5. Responsibility—knowing what is expected of you and not making excuses for poor performance
6. Respect—maintaining healthy habits for your body and having consideration for those around you
7. Enjoyment—make sure to include some fun in practice and during competition
8. Perseverance—the ability to give full effort regardless of the circumstances

Integrity: Be Honest

Integrity is the cornerstone of long-term success in sports. You can't shortcut the way to athletic excellence by cramming a week before competition or expecting a super boost from a hot new product. You have to apply sound principles and use reliable training techniques.

One of the main issues challenging the integrity of today's athlete is the use of so-called performance-enhancing drugs. Although some products may produce marginal short-term benefits in size and strength, their effect on overall performance is questionable (Ellender 2005). In spite of this, your competitors may be armed with a combination of anabolic steroids, growth hormones, and concentrated blood products. They may have little or no regard for how these products damage their health, and they rarely consider how it damages their self-image and self-esteem. The use of illegal, performance-enhancing drugs is not only unhealthy, it's cheating against your opponents and it's cheating yourself.

We'll see throughout this chapter how your self-image and self-confidence are an important part of your athletic foundation (Hardy 1992). When you cheat, you will eventually pay the price one way or another. The guilt will hang over your shoulders like an anchor. It will demoralize you when you've been beaten and rob you of the full appreciation of your victories. In the end, you only cheat yourself.

Fortunately, there is much more to being a successful athlete than taking harmful, ineffective chemicals (Greydanus 2002). This book is about developing the personal habits that result in superior athletic performance, so when all is said and done, whether you are winning bragging rights or gold medals, you can do so with complete satisfaction.

Preparedness: Be Ready

Most athletes will spend more time preparing than competing. Being ready isn't a natural talent; it's a choice. Even if you haven't been ready in the past, you can change this behavior in the future.

How do you become an athlete who is ready to practice and compete? Most of this book explores that question, but these are a few areas you'll want to pay attention to:

- Stay in shape
- Eat the right foods
- Stay hydrated
- Get enough rest
- Have the right equipment
- Know where you need to be and get there early
- Be prepared for the unexpected

It's your choice: be ready or start making up excuses for why you weren't.

Teamwork: Be a Team Player

A good team isn't just a bunch of talented players with the same jerseys. It's a cohesive group of players who can work together during good times and bad. It's easy to be a good teammate when your team is hot. Everyone is cheering and you're scoring big points. You're all working together, and your team seems invincible.

Meanwhile, on the losing side, the players are demoralized and blame each other for their poor performance. Unresolved conflicts are surfacing, and soon the team members will be at each other's throats. At this point, it doesn't matter how talented you are. If your team is not playing together, you're going to lose. Under these circumstances, team members have to pull together, support one another, and not get rattled. It starts with keeping your head up, projecting a positive attitude, and performing your best. You'll be surprised at how well you can control your opponent's momentum by not falling apart when times get tough. Being a good leader in these situations means helping to keep your teammates focused on the goal.

Being a good teammate is just as important during practice as it is during competition. Whether you compete individually or on a team, your training partners will push you to a level of performance that you won't achieve by yourself. Your teammates aren't only going to challenge your skills; they are the ones that will make the long, hard hours of practice enjoyable. The relationships you develop with your teammates will make the good times better and the hard times easier to endure.

Cox (1988, p.305–306) has outlined ten recommendations for developing team cohesion:

1. Get to know each other's responsibilities
2. Learn something personal about each player
3. Develop pride within subunits of large teams
4. Develop a feeling of ownership among players
5. Set team goals and take pride in their accomplishments
6. Learn your role and why it is important
7. Don't expect complete social tranquility
8. Avoid forming cliques
9. Develop team drills and lead-up games that encourage cooperation
10. Highlight your successes even if you lose a game or match

Adaptability: Be Flexible

Athletes have to practice and compete in a variety of circumstances and your attitude toward change will affect your performance. You might have to play a different position or compete during the hot part of the day. The one thing that you can count on is that things will change.

Even when they change, you always have a choice. You can get flustered or you can choose to adapt and commit to doing your best regardless of the circumstances. You can take it a step further and allow yourself to like the change. In fact, change can put you at an advantage if you've done your homework and are prepared to compete in a variety of circumstances. Don't forget that your thoughts and beliefs will affect your performance. So if it rains during your golf tournament, learn to love golfing in the rain.

Responsibility: Know Your Role

Responsibility means a great deal in sports, and like preparedness, it is not a natural talent but a choice. From covering your position to knowing the plays, being a responsible player means accepting your role on the team and not making excuses or blaming someone else for your poor performance. You can't change the wind speed, the temperature, or the referee. You can't blame your coach, your teammates, or your dog (unless, of course, you're into dogsled racing) for a poor performance. This is another great opportunity to take on a leadership role and be the one that makes it happen, so be prepared to carry your weight and a little more.

Respect: Show Compassion and Consideration

Respect starts with self-respect. This means making the choices that nurture your body, mind, and spirit. On the other hand, self-destructive choices such as drugs use, poor nutrition, or unhealthy habits will eventually rob you of your ability to perform at your best.

The inner strength and maturity that comes from self-respect will make it easier to respect the people around you. It's unfortunate to see any athlete, let alone a famous one, treat their opponents disrespectfully. Along with notoriety comes the responsibility to those that look up to you because of your ability. It's an obligation that comes with the territory and is the price of being a leader within your field. When all is said and done, the way you treat those around you, including your opponents, is truly a reflection of your own inner strength.

Enjoyment: Have Fun

Deciding to enjoy what you're doing can be one of the most important decisions that you'll ever make. The long hours of training and the pressures of competition can be exhausting. You don't have to wait for the pot of gold at the end. Go ahead and take advantage of the many sources of enjoyment along the way.

One way to avoid drudgery is to make it a point to have some fun before, during, and after practice. After all, keeping an upbeat attitude will help you relax, improve your performance, and limit the amount of energy that you spend on being nervous, stiff, and uptight. Not only is this important for practice, but it is also critical during those high-pressure moments while you are competing. Again, your state of mind will affect your performance, so staying loose and having fun is a smart way to deal with the pressures of competition.

Perseverance: Don't Give Up

If it was all fun we would have no trouble staying motivated but sometimes things can get ugly. You might get so far behind that it seems as though you don't stand a chance to come back. Yet we've all seen incredible comebacks and perseverance was the driving force behind each one. Some of the most exciting athletic performances have been come-from-behind victories. *Being behind is an opportunity to perform beyond the best of your abilities.* Quitting means giving up this opportunity.

Successful athletes aren't made overnight; it takes years of preparation and training. There will be plenty of tough times and every athlete will have to face losses, injuries, and rejection.

How do the athletes that survive find the motivation to press on? You'll want to know so you don't sink the next time you fall in the quicksand.

Motivation

Having established a solid foundation, you are ready to ask yourself several important questions: *What's motivating you? Why do you want to be an athlete, and why do you want to strive to be good at your sport?*

Since you are going to dedicate many long, hard hours to mastering your sport, you might as well try to understand what's driving you. The common things that motivate other athletes are listed below; you may want to think about how they apply to your situation:

- Enjoyment—the pure thrill of competition
- Skills development—improving the way you play the game
- Physical appearance—maintaining a solid body frame
- Stress management—keeping yourself healthy through exercise
- Financial gain—the opportunity for the elite athlete to earn a comfortable living
- Camaraderie—the friendships built by teamwork
- Notoriety and acceptance—developing an identity from being a member of a team
- Self-actualization—the feeling of accomplishment from success in the arena
- Entertainment—having an activity to anticipate
- Social skills development—how to communicate and work together as a team
- Intellectual challenge—finding the best strategy to beat a difficult opponent
- Self-discipline—the power of sticking to a routine

One way to get motivated is to set attainable yet challenging goals. Your short-term goals can serve as stepping stones to bigger and better achievements. For example, the short-term goal of improving your running speed and endurance can help you achieve your long-term goal of making the varsity soccer team. It's a good idea to set goals that are objective and easy to measure. Setting goals for strength and fitness are easy to monitor by measuring your performance on the track and in the weight room. For many athletes, the goal may just be to play the game, have some fun, and stay in shape. Regardless of your ambitions, the goals you set can help you prioritize your training and reward you with the self-satisfaction that comes with achievement.

Another way to think about motivation is whether it is internally or externally driven. Money and fame are significant external motivators, but don't lose sight of the big picture and let your ambitions overpower your ideals. There is no amount of money or fame that is worth compromising your standing with God, your relationships with the people you love, or your integrity. In the long run, the ideal way to keep performing at your best is to develop a powerful internal motivation by being committed to personal excellence and learning to enjoy and appreciate the gifts you have received.

In the purest sense, competitive sports are a way to bring out the best in human performance. Each athlete is doing their best to push the other athlete to the upper limits of their ability, and in the end, the best athlete is declared the winner.

The concept of doing your best and actualizing your potential is important because on your way to the top you'll need to challenge your skills by competing against tougher competitors. If the competition is challenging enough, they will teach you some painful lessons. If you are an athlete who can only focus on winning, taking an occasional beating can be devastating. On the other hand, if you can keep an eye on the big picture, it will be easier to recover and look forward to using the lessons you learned during your next event.

You can see why becoming a champion is not just about winning a championship; it's about staying motivated and having the mental perspective that will help you survive the preparation.

Monitor Your Thoughts

Have you ever wondered why so many baseball pitchers have trouble hitting the ball? Could there be some genetic reason that some pitchers can't even fake a good swing? I doubt it. It boils down to the belief that no one, including the pitcher, expects them to hit the ball. Since this is such a good example of how your mental perspective affects your performance let's take a moment to explore it.

The cognitive theory of psychology suggests that what you think has an effect on how you feel and behave. It challenges us to evaluate what we are thinking, whether it is true, and whether it's in our best interest. There are a number of beliefs that keep pitchers from being better hitters, and there are some good arguments that perpetuate these beliefs. After all, they have to focus on their pitching. You can also argue that since they aren't playing in every game, they get less experience at stepping up to the plate. Regardless, it's a historically accepted norm, and as long as they pitch well they are excused. They internalize the belief system, give up on batting practice, and step up to the plate with a lower expectation. The price, unfortunately, is that one out of nine hitters is a dud.

The challenge is to get the pitcher to step up to the plate with the expectation and full belief that he is going to hit the ball as well as anyone else. Now I know you're looking back at the cover to see if this book is about sports science or science fiction, but let's challenge this belief system because it illustrates some important principles that can help you improve many aspects of your performance.

First, let's establish that our pitcher—call him Joe—has all the necessary endowments to be able to hit the ball. His vision is okay, he has reasonable muscle development, and he has normal coordination. After all, he is a pitcher. Keep in mind that he doesn't need to be a big, powerful guy to hit a home run, let alone a base hit. From the mechanical perspective, all he has to do is to swing the bat hard enough to get a bat speed of 70 mph to generate enough power to send it out of the park (Adair 1994). With the right timing and body mechanics, a bat speed of 70 mph is well within the reach of most well-developed adult male athletes. In fact, Roger Maris hit home runs as well as anyone, and he weighed less than 200 pounds. It really comes down to timing, mechanics, and the belief that you're able to do it. You also need a lot of practice.

Think Positively

To get started, our pitcher is going to have to set aside all the negative commentary about hitting and replace them with positive thoughts. Joe will tell himself that he's going to be a hitter, that he looks forward to stepping up to the plate, and that he loves the sound of the bat hitting the ball. He can take it a step further. He can argue that he has an advantage because he knows more about pitching and has a better idea of what the pitcher is going to throw. As part of his goal to become a hitter, Joe will study the hitters around him, ask them questions, and step up to the plate with them. Hitting will become an important part of Joe's training.

Before we get too far into the example, I want to take a quick moment to put the concept of positive thinking into perspective. Obviously, you can't just think your way into becoming a good athlete; you have to put your heart into it and do the work. It's like turning on the light at your desk. It won't get your homework done, but it will make it a lot easier to see what you're doing. Without some optimism about your ability to succeed, it will be hard to get started and even harder to keep going.

Positive thinking has another limitation: it will help achieve your true potential, but it won't turn you into something that you aren't capable of becoming. Even though optimism can help you break down barriers and improve your performance, you need to maintain a healthy degree of realism to keep you from getting disappointed.

In other words, for our example, positive thinking will not make Joe a better hitter unless he practices. It's clearly helpful to be optimistic because if he thought negatively and believed that practicing was useless, he might as well go lie on the couch and eat cheese puffs. It's like closing the door and turning off the lights when you have to do that homework. You'll never get your work done. If Joe thinks positively and works hard, he will come closer to achieving his potential as a hitter, but he is going to have to maintain some degree of realism. No matter how hard he tries, we all have limits and we need to come to terms with them when we reach them.

Now that we have established that a positive outlook can help you get started, what do you do if you don't seem to be making progress? Joe has to keep in mind that he will be fighting an uphill battle because even after years of practice, the best hitters only get hits every one out of three times they bat. Joe's going to have to develop a long-term perspective so that he doesn't fall into the trap of believing he can't do it when he fails nine times out of ten. At this rate of failure, it is hard to stay motivated unless you realize that success is a long-term project. *When you are trying to improve a difficult skill, you need to remember that success is not measured by your performance, but by your level of motivation.*

We all have areas that need improvement. When you are evaluating a problem in some aspect of your performance (or your life), there are some points to consider.

Start by looking at what you are thinking and then ask yourself whether it's helpful. Helpful is a key word here because even negative thoughts can be helpful. For example, you might think that you aren't in good enough shape to compete. If this negative thought is true, it can motivate you to get in shape. In this situation, the thought you don't want to carry around is: "I'll never get in good enough shape to achieve my goal." The other thoughts you don't want to ignore are messages about thirst, heat, pain, and fatigue. If you ignore these thoughts you can end up dehydrated, overheated, or injured.

Here are some ideas to get you started:

- What are you telling yourself?
  - I can't do it.
  - I am a specialist in a different aspect of the game so I don't have to do it.
  - I've never been able to do it.
  - I'm not good at it.
  - I'm not tall, fast, strong, coordinated, or quick enough.
  - I don't have the right equipment.

- What are you visualizing?
- What are your feelings and how does it feel to perform this particular task?
- Is there a *true* genetic or permanent physical disability that is preventing success?
- Are your past experiences and performances an absolute predictor of future performances?
- What is your long-term goal, and what does the big picture look like?

Can you:
- Change negative thoughts into positive ones?
- Imagine yourself doing it right?
- Feel yourself doing it correctly?
- See yourself recovering the next time you do it incorrectly?

How can you back up your new thoughts with action and experience? What can you do to become the expert?

- Ask questions
- Watch the experts
- Get coaching
- Keep trying
- Practice
- Watch videos of yourself performing the task
- Give yourself a break if you are getting frustrated
- See chapter six for a more in-depth discussion of how to improve your skills

When dealing with team issues, consider asking your teammates what they are thinking. Then you can engage their support and input on the solution. Practice the winning move with them so that they can feel confident in your abilities. Finally, don't forget to thank them and appreciate them for their support.

For example, if your sport is basketball, these principles can be applied to learning team skills, like how to make extra passes to get high-percentage shots or learning individual skills, like how to improve one's free throw percentage.

Manage Your Stress

Since too much stress will make it hard to keep a positive mental perspective, you'll want to have a good understanding of how stress affects you. In *The New*

Toughness Training for Sports, James Loehr does an excellent job of reviewing stress management for athletes. One of the key points is that the right amount of stress balanced by the right amount of recovery makes you stronger. With this in mind, it's not surprising that the athletes who consistently perform at the upper levels of their abilities will take advantage of every opportunity to recover. They are the experts at maintaining and regaining their composure in situations where other athletes lose theirs.

If you want to learn how to manage your stress, you'll want to understand how stress makes you stronger. Let's take the example of an average runner, Elizabeth, who's just decided that she wants to run a marathon. She's been running three miles every other day for the past few months, so her body has already adapted to running but not at the level of running a marathon. To get ready, she needs to gradually acclimate to higher levels of stress so that come race day, her body will be fully adapted. If she takes on too much too soon, she'll risk injury and exhaustion. On the other hand, if she increases her mileage too slowly, she won't be ready.

Fortunately, she knows that increasing her mileage by more than 10% per week is associated with a higher rate of injury. She's planning to slowly increase her mileage (stress) over a five-month period to get to a level where she can run forty miles in a week.

The training part is straightforward, but what many athletes fail to consider is that the way you recover is just as important as how hard you train. It's while she is recovering that her bones and muscles are actually getting stronger. In addition, Elizabeth is thinking about the other types of stress that she will encounter during her training for the marathon. These include heat, chafing, and blistering, as well as maintaining adequate hydration and nutrition.

To get used to running in the heat, Elizabeth is going to train in the afternoon when it's warmer. She will make time to drink and eat properly and will rest at least two days per week. She'll be sure to relax and spend some time with her boyfriend on her days off.

Some athletes don't believe that their personal lives affect their athletic performance. Although there is no doubt that heavy training and competition is stressful, when you add stressful life events to the mix, the results can be overwhelming. High levels of personal stress can increase your risk of injury, and the chemicals that circulate through your body while you are stressed can have far-reaching effects that include decreased immunity and even decreased peripheral vision (Ahern 1997).

Let's look at some examples of the stress an athlete faces during practice and competition.

Physical stress

- Musculoskeletal stress: the stress on your bones, ligaments, joints, tendons, and muscles
- Aerobic stress: the stress on your cardiovascular and muscular systems to deliver and utilize oxygen at high levels
- Anaerobic stress: the stress on your cardiovascular and muscular systems to perform when there is not enough oxygen to meet the demand. Examples are sprinting and other activities that require rapid, intense bursts of energy
- Environmental stress: heat, cold, humidity, wind, sun, and altitude
- Nutritional stress: maintaining adequate hydration, electrolyte balance (changes in sodium and potassium levels can decrease performance), caloric balance, and optimal intake of vitamins and minerals

Mental stress

- You'll need to stay focused and upbeat when your body is exhausted and the crowd is heckling you.
- You'll have to remember the mechanical aspects of your sport such as technique, strategies, plays, and rules.
- You'll need to make the right decisions regarding strategies, finances, teams, equipment, and coaches.

We've already reviewed some of the approaches to dealing with mental stress earlier in this chapter. They include being prepared, knowing your sport, and staying committed to good principles. You can also use your cognitive techniques to keep you focused and in the right state of mind.

Emotional stress

Examples of emotional stress include:

- Dealing with injuries, losses, and unmet expectations
- Dealing with the stress of success

- Dealing with the interpersonal pressures associated with long hours of practice, traveling, and financial worries
- Dealing with issues related to criticism, anger, and fear

Dealing with criticism, anger, or nervousness can have a huge effect on how well you perform. Let's spend some time exploring each one of these emotional stressors and how you can develop strategies for coping with them.

The best coaches can push you to levels of performance that you can't imagine. On the other hand, they can rip you to pieces if you're too sensitive to their criticism. Learning to deal with criticism, and sometimes abuse, is an essential art that every athlete needs to develop. Before we go on, I want to make one point very clear: I *do not* advocate abusive language or behavior in any way, shape, or form. On the other hand, I've been around long enough to know that from time to time, even the best coaches will lose their temper and utter some unforgivable remark. Although most of these remarks are unfounded, you don't want to let them damage your self-esteem.

Since you will definitely interact with obnoxious coaches (and other people, like teachers, drill sergeants, and bosses), you might as well be prepared. This is where a solid sense of identity and self-worth can keep you thinking calmly and clearly in the most intimidating situations.

The first thing to keep in mind is that most of these interactions are driven by frustration and they have little, if any, basis in truth. It's probably not even about you so try not to take it personally. You have to realize that the perpetrator is just blowing off steam, and your goal is to keep from getting burned. If there is some truth to the matter, take a mental note and commit to doing your best to correct it. Think of the criticism as an opportunity to take corrective action. It's okay to disregard the static around the message and use the cognitive techniques you've already learned to avoid replaying the negative comment in your head.

When you encounter a hostile situation, think of it as an opportunity to practice staying cool, calm, and collected in the face of anger and intimidation. It's similar to any other training you do: the tougher the challenge, the better you get.

One of the first things to keep in mind is the importance of not appearing rattled or intimidated because most obnoxious people will behave like sharks when they smell blood. If they see that you're vulnerable, they'll make you the target of their next feeding frenzy. Here are some suggestions for how to respond to criticism:

- Go about your business with no specific response. Most of these interactions do not warrant a response and at times responding may lead to an escalation in the level of anger.
- Maintain good posture, take a deep breath, and think "calm."
- Delay your response until after the person has had a moment to cool down.
- Acknowledge any truthful part of the message and your intention to improve. Then follow it with action.

It is important to understand that there are limits to abuse and that we all have an obligation to stand up against abuse when it gets out of hand. If you are a young athlete, you may want to talk it over with a parent, teacher, or counselor so that you have the necessary support to take the appropriate action.

Coaching our youth is a huge responsibility and most coaches are able to combine their knowledge, experience, and personal fortitude to provide an excellent service to their athletes. The majority of coaches are well-meaning, hardworking, underpaid people who give their time and energy to help young athletes have fun, improve their performance, and become better people. Even with the best intentions, some coaches can fall into various degrees of abusive behaviors when confronted by situations that they aren't prepared to handle. In some cases, it is more than a transient vulnerability that is rapidly recognized and corrected; it's a pattern of systematic intent to exploit their power and position. It's difficult to address this ugly side of sports, but ignoring it won't make it go away.

Crossing the Line

When do the coach's actions cross the line from healthy motivation to harmful abuse? To address this question, we need to take a step back and look at the big picture. What are our goals and what are we trying to teach the athlete? Many of the lessons that athletes need to learn are physically and emotionally demanding and developing an appropriate level of toughness is part of the lesson. Hopefully, our goal is to contribute to the healthy personal and athletic development of our young athlete and not the modeling, acceptance, and normalization of abusive behaviors.

Our first challenge is to assess the athlete's capabilities as well as their limitations so that the coach and the athlete can set realistic performance goals. It makes no sense to expect a little leaguer to perform at the level of a professional. Regardless of whether it is coming from the athlete, the parent, or the coach, unrealistic expectations are a frequent cause of frustration and disappointment.

Having determined realistic goals, the coach needs to develop a framework of appropriate feedback including a disciplinary system of rewards, limit setting, and consequences. The type of feedback and discipline vary depending on the athlete's needs and the coach's style, but some approaches are clearly better than others. The best approach values the athlete's well-being as much as it does winning.

Abuse begins when the athlete's well-being is not part of the formula. Frequently it is unintentional and has its roots in frustration as well as lack of experience and training. In this circumstance, minor breaches in judgment and behavior are forgivable as long as they are isolated and corrected. Unfortunately, some coaches fail to see the error of their ways and continue their approach even in the face of repeated warnings. We need to recognize that there is an unacceptable level of systematic abuse by coaches in all levels of sports. It involves emotional, physical, and sexual abuse and the results are devastating. We need to increase awareness so that we can develop guidelines and programs to prevent this problem.

Setting these guidelines is complicated by expectations, feedback, and disciplinary actions that vary with the athlete's age and level of competition. Again, it makes no sense to slap a $5,000 fine on a little leaguer for showing up late to practice. Regardless of age, though, some behavior patterns are just not acceptable.

Systematic emotional abuse manifests itself in many ways, and it is frequently the cornerstone of subsequent physical and sexual abuse. The patterns of emotional abuse include, but are not limited to, unrealistic expectations, excessive negative feedback, and unfair disciplinary actions.

The emotionally abusive coach frequently yells, personalizes, blames, and scapegoats the players. The relentless onslaught of negative feedback and punishment creates a sense of hopelessness and low self-esteem in the victimized player. Granted, some coaching situations are conducive to yelling because of the distance separating the players on the field. It's the inappropriate yelling combined with negative commentary about the athlete as a person as opposed to their performance that does the harm. Some coaches like to isolate players and repeatedly humiliate them in front of their peers with name-calling and negative slurs. They will also encourage other teammates to harass the victimized player as a way of developing a sense of superiority amongst selected players.

Some emotionally abusive coaches use excessive physical punishment to discipline and humiliate their players. We're not talking about running an extra lap or doing ten push-ups as penance for an error. Some coaches will run their players and their teams ragged as a punishment for poor performance. In other circumstances, the coaches will encourage the team to physically abuse a player who is not performing up to a standard.

It may seem easy to detect and correct this type of abuse, but many athletes are hesitant to speak up or even quit because they fear retaliation and social isolation by their peers. In a win-at-any-cost environment, it's easy to label the athlete that speaks up as a wimp, and the involvement of teammates in the abuse can create a code of silence among the favored players.

Physical abuse of the athlete isn't limited to punishment, and at times it may be rationalized as a way of making the athlete tougher or even as a way of rewarding a talented player. Coaches who don't understand or refuse to accept the dangers of overtraining develop a "survival of the fittest" attitude and run their athletes into the ground during the process. Some coaches will place talented athletes on a pedestal, and in their drive to win they will expect the athlete to play at an unsustainable level until the athlete is injured or burns out.

From the surface, these subtle, manipulative approaches to abuse are harder to recognize because the coach uses rewards, praise, and favoritism to get something from the athlete. The athlete starts to believe that they owe the coach something, and they are afraid to let the coach down.

Regardless of the method, athletes who are physically and emotionally worn down are highly vulnerable to other forms of abuse, including sexual abuse and substance abuse. Substance abuse can include "performance-enhancing" drugs as well as other forms of drugs and alcohol. Athletes desperate to improve their performance are more likely to risk their health and integrity by using steroids, whether it is their own idea or through the encouragement of a coach or teammate. In a similar fashion, athletes having difficulty coping are more likely to use drugs or alcohol as a maladaptive way of managing their stress. This kind of behavior leads to a vicious cycle in the wrong direction.

The sexual abuse of athletes is more common than people care to admit. The spectrum spans from sexually explicit verbal abuse to various forms of rape. The majority of victims are teenage girls and young women, but they can include males as well. The coach is usually male and takes advantage of their age, experience, and the frequent opportunities for physical closeness, as well as the power and trust associated with their position to manipulate their vulnerable victims. Teenage girls are particularly susceptible because they quickly confuse their hormonally driven infatuation with "true love." Their lack of experience combined with their precocious need to appear grown-up leaves them gullible, impressionable, and terribly vulnerable.

Once the stage is set, the male perpetrator just has to show up on the scene and with a few smiles and winks, their victims will be eating out of his hands. From the surface, the scene can appear confusing because the young girl becomes so wrapped up in her infatuation; she appears to be the one making the moves. The perpetrator is quick to capitalize on this confusion by blaming the victim and pathetically hiding his lack of fortitude and conscience behind the young girl's advances. Since they know their actions are wrong, the "coach" frequently encourages the victim to keep the relationship a secret, thereby adding to the drama and romance that many young girls find so attractive. Being completely blinded by infatuation, it may take months or years for the young girl to understand that their coach is nothing but a smooth-talking rapist who should be exposed as such as soon as possible.

Unlike other forms of rape where the rapist uses physical strength or a weapon to overcome the victim's defenses, this type of rapist exploits experience and social power. They abuse the trust placed in them by the athlete, their parents, and their community to manipulate a naïve and essentially defenseless victim.

Although this form of abuse occurs most commonly between young male coaches and teenage girls, the perpetrators can include male and female coaches, trainers, family members, and even senior athletes within a team or league. Some perpetrators will even take advantage of the adolescent's common confusion about gender roles and sexuality to manipulate them into same-sex abuse. The athlete needs to understand this is not a normal coach-athlete relationship by any stretch of the imagination.

If you are not yet thoroughly disgusted, we still need to address the problem of outright forcible rape in sports. Twenty-five percent of the women in our society will be sexually assaulted by the time they are eighteen years old. The sporting world offers no immunity to this disease. The range of abuse includes everything from date rape to gang rape. The perpetrators are friends, acquaintances, teammates, strangers, coaches, trainers, family members, and members of your school's team or the opposing team. Sometimes they will go to great lengths to gain everyone's trust and confidence, and they will use their power and position to discourage the victim from speaking out. The horror of this kind of violent cruelty defies further expression.

If you are starting to feel a little apprehensive or even paranoid, you need to be. Prevention starts with awareness and education. As an athlete, you need to be aware of your vulnerabilities as well as the warning signs and patterns of abuse. You can always go to your parents, a teacher, the principal, or a trusted friend to discuss your concerns and to get support for taking the appropriate action. As adults, we need to develop guidelines and education for appropriate coaching procedures as well as systems for independent monitoring of athletics programs. We need to establish a way for athletes that are being abused to speak up without fear of retaliation. Finally, we need to develop a system for identifying and disciplining abusers, particularly repetitive abusers.

Don't Get Angry...

Anger is an emotional response that comes from both internal and external frustration. Externally, it can come from the perception of being treated unfairly. Internally, it will present itself as self-directed anger from not meeting your expectations and having to face the fact that you aren't perfect.

Along with the unpleasant emotional sensations that come with anger, you'll experience important physiological changes *that will impair your performance*. The fight-or-flight response will pump adrenaline through your body, increasing your heart rate and blood pressure. Your muscles will become tense, and it will be harder to concentrate. Getting yourself keyed up may be of value if your sport requires a short burst of energy with little or no technique. However, most sports require some degree of pacing along with significant attention to technique. Athletes who have to explode with energy, such as sprinters and weight lifters, are focused on good timing and proper execution of their skills. Even fighting, which would seem to capitalize on anger, is dominated by strategy, technique, and pacing.

From the other side of the field, it looks even worse for the angry competitor. Seeing your opponent get frustrated can be motivating because it's evidence that you are getting under his skin (Hackfort 1996). You may want to keep this in mind when you are getting frustrated, because the last thing you want to do is to motivate your opponent.

Angry athletes have another major problem to deal with: burnout. Constantly revving yourself with anger is a sure way to lose the enjoyment of your sport.

When you start to feel angry, you need to put your cognitive skills to work. It's not that you always want to avoid anger because in certain situations some degree of anger may be perfectly appropriate.

On the other hand, you probably don't want to let your anger get to the point that you start to behave in a way that you'll regret. It's up to you to take a moment to evaluate the stimulus and *choose the best response*. In sports, getting angry is usually not the best response.

Let's look at some examples.

A spectator insults you or your team. The spectator is the one with the problem, and as long as they stay in the stands, there is no significant threat.

The referee makes a bad call. Referees make many calls. Most are correct, and the incorrect ones tend to balance each other out. Under most circumstances, one bad call won't make you or break you, so there is no significant threat.

You make an error. You're not perfect and both sides will make errors. As long as you don't make too many errors, there is no significant threat.

Another player pushes you after the play is over. The other player is upset about you scoring another point, and although he pushed you, the threat to you is minimal.

Frequently, the initial perception of someone yelling at you, disagreeing with you, or trying to intimidate you may seem threatening, but if you stop to think about it, there really isn't much danger unless someone physically attacks you. Even if someone pushes you, they usually won't hurt you. Once you realize that you aren't in danger, it will be easier for you to take a moment to consider the best response.

Keep in mind that even if the threat is real, you can take advantage of the calm response because your opponent will perceive it as a sign of your inner strength and confidence. Taking this approach will catch your adversary by surprise and motivate them to reconsider their approach.

Let's look at some options for responding to offensive or hostile stimuli.

You can fly off the handle, yell and scream, jump up and down, get in their face, push them, and then throw a few punches. The result of this approach will be getting kicked out of the game, hurting someone, or if your opponent is a tough guy, you might be the one with the injuries. It may have worked once or twice, so you continue using this approach even though it may get you into deeper trouble. Whether you're on or off the field, the hostile option usually makes the situation worse. You may want to look at other options.

Another way is to go about your business with no specific response. Whether you feel threatened or not, this can be a very effective way to deal with the situation. The best response to an obscene phone call continues to be no response. The obnoxious person is trying to feel a sense of power by rattling your cage. By not responding, you're showing them that you are strong enough to not be rattled by their huffing and puffing.

You can also just laugh and shake your head. This approach is particularly valuable when you've made a mistake, and you're angry with yourself. A little humor can lighten your spirit and help you get in the right state of mind to continue competing. You can occasionally use humor when you are dealing with other people's hostility, but you need to practice some diplomacy or they might get even angrier.

You can also get a better understanding of the person's concern and let them know that you've gotten the message by taking the corrective action. For example, if you've been elbowing your opponent, then stop elbowing them.

These are useful ways to deal with the anger of the moment, but what about the anger that you carry around for longer periods? I'm talking about that anger that hangs around well past the event that triggered it. It's unpleasant, self-defeating, and unhealthy. You need to take some time to think it over, and once you've decided that you've done everything within your reasonable control, you need to just let it go and start your recovery. Yes—get over it and move on because it won't do you any good to carry it around. We'll be talking more about the importance of developing a variety of ways to recover from the everyday stress that you'll experience in sports and in life.

You can prevent hostile responses from other players by establishing yourself as an athlete who treats other players fairly and respectfully. If you routinely treat the other players respectfully, they might be less likely to attack you if you accidentally step on their toes. On the other hand, if you have a reputation for being obnoxious, your opponents will be waiting to punish you the moment you step out of line.

Monitor Your Level of Excitement

Like being angry, being scared has both a cognitive and emotional dimension. The mental component is characterized by worry—those intrusive thoughts about what might happen in a variety of future circumstances. As the threat appears more realistic, your body pours out the chemicals that prepare you to fight or take flight. You get a little shaky, your heart starts to pound, and your muscles start to become tense.

Facing a challenge or taking a risk is part of the fun of being in sports. The thrill of dropping onto a steep ski slope or walking into an arena full of cheering fans can excite you and improve your performance. It's when you believe that the ski slope might be too steep or that your opponent is too tough that your thoughts become negative, and your level of anxiety becomes counterproductive. Sports scientists use the term *arousal* to describe this spectrum of mental and physical responses. The response can range from frank boredom to excitement and even to outright terror.

Most top-notch athletes are able to monitor their level of arousal, and they have a variety of effective tools to combat excessive fear, anxiety, or boredom. Since maintaining a healthy level of excitement can help you perform at your best, you'll want to spend a moment reviewing the spectrum of arousal and how it affects your performance. Once you understand this, you can start to monitor your level of excitement and develop a variety of ways to deal with anxiety-provoking situations.

When you enter a competitive situation, your perceptions about the outcome and its potential effect can take several forms.

You can be highly confident that you will succeed and survive the competition intact. Being overly confident can lead to lack of arousal, boredom, and careless mistakes.

You can be confident about your ability to win while still maintaining some degree of caution about the situation. In most sporting situations, it's helpful to be confident and optimistic, but it is also important to maintain some degree of excitement so that you don't become bored and inattentive.

You can be uncertain about your ability to succeed and survive the competition intact. Uncertainty is one of the main sources of anxiety, and it may lead to excessive worrying, hesitation, and difficulty in focusing. Being overly anxious is an unpleasant sensation and prolonged anxiety can lead to fatigue and dissatisfaction with your sport.

You can also think that you will be defeated and probably sustain a significant injury or setback in your career. Fear is the best word to describe this situation. As your worries become reality, your level of tension increases. The adrenaline pumping through your blood will give you a short burst of energy at the expense of technique and endurance. In competition, persistent fear can be debilitating.

Clearly, the best situation is the second one. However, fear has a way of sneaking into your consciousness. You'll want to develop a variety of ways to keep the jitters in check so that they don't upset your performance. They include the following:

1. *Develop self-confidence and a core belief that you can do it.* This starts with your thoughts but needs to be followed up with hard work and preparation. Developing the character traits and values that we discussed earlier in this chapter can help you develop a sense of worthiness about athletic competition.

2. *Learn to monitor your level of arousal/anxiety.* Self-awareness is an endowment that we all can develop with practice. It means being on the lookout for worrisome thoughts and monitoring your body for signs of tension and overexcitement. These include accelerated heart rate, shallow breathing, stiffness, and tremors.

3. *Replace worrisome thoughts with positive ones.* You can do this by putting your cognitive techniques to work. A good place to start is to realize that worrying will not help your performance and that being relaxed is the best option.

4. *Learn to calm your physical and mental response to anxiety/arousal.* Meditation is a proven method of calming your mind and body. You can learn to relax in a quiet setting, and once you've developed some experience you can apply the basics in a variety of settings. The first step for relaxation is to find a comfortable position and begin to change your breathing pattern to a slower, deeper cycle because slow, deep breaths will initiate a relaxation response. Once your breathing is on a good cycle you can focus on muscle relaxation. There are varieties of methods, but a simple one is to focus on your feet, tightening your muscles then relaxing them by shaking them out. Gradually move up your body and pay close attention to areas of muscle tension. As you proceed, you'll learn to identify tense areas in your body and to relax them at will. Once your body is relaxed, you can begin to focus on your mind.

Many approaches to relaxation include visualizations of soothing thoughts and scenes, but what if you are stuck in a noisy gym? Not a problem. You can learn to relax by expanding your awareness and focusing on all the nonvisual sensations around you, including sounds and tactile sensations. In this setting, instead of the noise and commotion becoming a problem, it actually becomes your ticket to relaxation. The key is to relax and see if you can take in all the sounds and sensations. You'll notice that you will pass through a variety of stages of relaxation and that, with practice, you can learn to adjust your level of relaxation with ease. Once you have developed some mastery over these techniques, you can apply them to a variety of settings including the pregame jitters as well as clutch situations.

5. *Don't get too relaxed.* Boredom will lead to careless mistakes, and even though it's nice to be relaxed and confident, you don't want to fall into the trap of taking your success for granted. You can avoid boredom by having fun, exciting the crowd, and maintaining a healthy degree of respect for your opponent. You can stay physically alert by moving around, stretching, and staying on your toes.

One of the other causes of under-arousal is fatigue and exhaustion. When you get tired, you won't be able to react as quickly, and it will be harder to go the extra distance. We'll see how you can minimize the amount of fatigue that you experience by doing the right kind of training and developing good nutritional habits.

6. *Develop a support system.* You can develop a better sense of security by surrounding yourself by people that care about you for being the person that you are. Knowing that they'll be there for you, win or lose, will lessen some of the outcome pressures that many athletes experience.

7. *Work with a safety net.* Trapeze artists can focus on what they are doing if they don't have to worry about hitting the ground at a hundred miles an hour. Having a safety net helps them stay relaxed and allows them the freedom to soar to greater heights. You can develop this sense by having a support system, a variety of interests, and a backup plan.

8. *Stay focused on the task at hand.* By staying focused on what you're doing, you'll do less worrying about some future situations that may never arise. Staying focused is a skill that requires practice. When you get up to bat, try to stay focused on hitting the ball and not your batting average, who's watching you, or what they're going to think if you strike out.

9. *Put yourself in God's hands and then do your best.* Keeping an eye on the big picture will help you keep your worries and fears in their proper perspective.

10. *Learn to recover.* We'll explore this in greater detail in the next few pages.

Learn to Recover: Maintaining Your Best Performance State

As you already know, the way that you recover from the stress of training and competition is just as important as how hard you train. Pushing yourself to the edge of your ability is physically and mentally exhausting, and it's during the recovery phase that you have an opportunity to regain your strength. If you want to perform at your best, you'll need to be an expert at recovering.

Being able to recover doesn't just apply to what you do off the field; it's an essential skill for practice and competition. In his book, James Loehr noted that athletes with long-term staying power have a superior ability to recover on or off the field. During practice and competition they use every opportunity to refocus and bring themselves to what he describes as an ideal performance state. This is "simply the optimal state of physiological and psychological arousal for performing at your peak. [Athletes] are most likely to experience ideal performance state and perform at their best when they feel confident, relaxed and calm, energized with positive emotion, challenged, focused and alert, automatic and instinctive, and ready for fun and enjoyment" (Loehr 1994).

Get in the Zone

Athletes who have achieved an optimal mental state have described exceptional ability as well as altered sensations and perceptions. These observations are difficult to quantify from a scientific perspective but have been reported by athletes across a variety of cultures. Michael Murphy and Rhea White have explored many of these reports in their book *In the Zone*. Some of these altered sensations are:

- Altered sense of time and space
- Unusual strength and speed
- Decreased pain sensation
- Exceptional focus
- Increased awareness
- Improved vision and hearing
- Calm and well-being
- Weightlessness
- Intuition
- Automaticity
- Performing instinctively
- Awe and ecstasy

Susan Jackson (1996) from the University of Queensland in Australia studied a group of elite athletes representing a variety of sports and confirmed that many of the athletes experienced a "flow" state that includes nine characteristics described by Csikszentmihalyi. These include:

1. A balance between the athlete's skill and the task being performed
2. A merging of action and awareness where the activity becomes almost automatic
3. A sense of goals being clearly set in advance so that the athlete knows what they have to do
4. Feedback becomes clear and unambiguous with everything going like clockwork
5. Complete focus and concentration on the task at hand with heightened awareness of the important aspects surrounding the athlete
6. An automatic and effortless sense of control
7. A loss of self-consciousness where the athlete develops a feeling of oneness with the environment
8. An altered sense of time
9. A heightened sense of enjoyment

Practice Your Mental State

Clearly, it would be great to be able to achieve and maintain this type of mental state, but the stress of intense practice and competition can make you anxious, tired, and distracted. The result is that you are not in the optimal physical, mental, or emotional condition to compete. This is when you need to take the opportunity to refocus by doing a quick self-assessment during every break in the action. You can improve your ability to recover by developing the following habits:

- Learn to monitor your breathing, heart rate, and muscle tension
- Maintain good posture
- Learn to excite the crowd and your teammates
- Give yourself positive messages
- Maintain adequate hydration, nutrition, and body temperature
- Enjoy yourself
- Stay focused on the task at hand
- Tune out negative internal and external commentary
- Practice turning on and maintaining your ideal performance state

It's equally important to develop a variety of ways to recover outside of training and competition. Your approach to recovery can range from being fully passive to very active, as Table 1.1 shows.

Most of these are self-explanatory. The important point is to make your hard work as fun as possible and then balance it with plenty of rest and recovery. As it is, you're going to be spending many hours perfecting your skills, so go ahead and enjoy it as much as you can.

	Recovery	
Passive	Active	
Prayer	Enjoying a different sport	
Listening to music	Yoga exercises	
Taking a hot bath	Dancing	
Massage	Learn something new	
Sleeping	Walking and hiking	
Eating a good meal	Swimming	
Watching a movie	Teaching	
Reading a book	Traveling	

Table 1.1. Ways to recover.

As the competition gets tougher, the competitors are always going to be talented. They're going to train just as hard as you will, maybe harder. You, on the other hand, are going to train smarter. With the right mental attitude, you'll train and compete with the edge that'll make you the better competitor.

Now that you've been introduced to the mental part of the game you're ready to start exploring how to optimize your physical fitness. At the top, it's not the most gifted athlete that wins; it's the one who is mentally and physically ready to compete.

CHAPTER 2

Nutrition

Think of your diet as part of your training program because what you eat and drink will affect your strength and endurance. Furthermore, the food that you eat will play an important role in the prevention of acute illnesses and chronic diseases. Don't let a weak nutritional foundation keep you from achieving your potential as an athlete.

The field of sports nutrition is full of controversy and conflicting advice, primarily because some opinions are based on half-baked science and financial incentive. Because you're likely going to be bombarded by a million different products and schemes, you might want to have a basic understanding of how to tell the difference between what works and what doesn't.

Be Skeptical

The first thing to keep in mind is that the nutritional supplement business is a billion-dollar industry and there are plenty of people who want to make a profit from your desire to get a competitive edge. The one thing you can count on is that the majority of the "performance enhancement" products that you see out there contain more hype than substance, so be skeptical.

In that case, how do you decide if a product is good for you? The first level of evidence is anecdotal or testimonial. You might find a well-known athlete that swears by Product X. The world champion may appear on the cover claiming that his success is due to the use of Product X. Unfortunately, even if our world champion is being honest, you can't be sure that his success is due to Product X until it has been systematically tested. From a scientific perspective, endorsements that lack accompanying measures to prove the claims of the product are close to worthless.

There are a number of factors, including the placebo effect, which can make it hard to know if a product is both safe and effective. We know that if someone believes a fake pill (placebo) contains an active ingredient, a significant number of people who take the placebo experience the preconceived effect. Your mind is so powerful that if you believe that something will happen, you will believe that something has happened. The more subjective the effects, such as "I feel better" or "I've been cleansed of toxins," the more likely that you will realize the effect by just thinking you do.

Even objectively measured results can be affected by the *placebo effect*. If you were to give a group of athletes a pill that they believed would make them taller, then a substantial number of the athletes would think they were taller. They could even measure themselves to be taller because they might stand more erect when being measured, or they might actually be taller because they grew. Never mind that their growth had nothing to do with the fake pill and happened because they were going to grow anyway! As you can see, a lot of factors affect the results of a study.

In an effort to try to counteract the placebo effect, scientists have developed a new system. In this system, the subjects are first matched for as many variables as possible. To get as uniform a group as possible, researchers try to match factors like age, sex, nutritional status, height, and weight. The subjects are then given the active ingredient and the control group is given the placebo. During the entire study period, neither the subjects nor the investigators know who is getting the real thing and who is getting the placebo.

At the end of the initial study period, the results are measured. The group that was given the active ingredient is then given the placebo, and the placebo group is given the active ingredient. The results are measured again at the end of the second study period, and then they are tabulated. Once all the information is collected, the investigators are allowed to know who was getting what product so they can see if there was a significant difference between the groups.

Again, even this method is not foolproof, and there are a number of factors that can bias the results of any study. For this reason, it's important to wait for the results of reputable, independent researchers to see if they can get similar results.

Finally, before you put anything in your body you have to ask yourself if it's safe. The safety issue can take years to evaluate because it takes time to know about the possible long-term side effects for any new product.

As you can see, trying to decide if the latest fad is going to turn you into a super athlete isn't easy. The good news is that you don't need to spend much time or money looking for the secret formula because just about everything that's out there is snake oil dressed up in a high-tech suit. To make things worse, some athletes become so preoccupied with putting chemicals into their bodies that they forget to eat properly. You, on the other hand, are going to get better results by focusing your energy on getting the right nutrition.

Well then, what do you need from a nutritional perspective? Let's start with the time-tested nutritional basic: food. The food that you eat contains six major components: carbohydrates, proteins, fats, vitamins, minerals, and water. You'll want to have a basic understanding about each of these food components so that you can be sure that you are getting the best nutrients.

Get Your Carbs

Carbohydrates are the primary fuel source for athletic activity. They come in two main varieties, simple and complex. Simple carbohydrates consist of a single sugar molecule (monosaccharides) or two sugar molecules combined (disaccharides). Examples of monosaccharides include glucose, fructose, and galactose.

Keep in mind that you're already familiar with some of these sugars. Maltose is the major component of malt, sucrose is table sugar, and lactose is the form of carbohydrate found in milk. With the exception of those who are lactose intolerant, most people easily absorb carbohydrates and convert them to glucose, the major fuel source. People with lactose intolerance have trouble breaking down the lactose in milk and develop diarrhea if they consume this form of carbohydrate.

Complex carbohydrates are glucose molecules that are attached to each other in long chains. They come in a variety of shapes and sizes and some are digestible while others are not. Digestible complex carbohydrates are called starches, and you can find them in breads, potatoes, pastas, and rice. Many sports nutrition products contain intermediate-sized carbohydrates called maltodextrins. They are typically made from cornstarch through a process that breaks the starch into smaller chains of carbohydrate.

Indigestible complex carbohydrates are called *fiber*, and although your body doesn't absorb them, they keep your intestines working normally and play a role in the prevention of a variety of diseases.

Once you absorb a carbohydrate, your body will convert it to glucose so that it can be transported to your cells via your blood stream. One of the first steps in absorbing glucose occurs as your pancreas senses a rise in your blood glucose and starts to produce *insulin*. The faster your glucose level rises, the more insulin your pancreas releases. It's with the help of insulin that your cells can absorb glucose for energy production.

Some carbohydrates are rapidly absorbed and cause a large release of insulin from your pancreas. That's not so bad until you consider that your insulin will outlast the quick blast of glucose, and it will continue to drive your blood glucose levels below their optimal range. As your blood glucose goes down, you'll start to feel less energetic. To complicate matters, insulin will block the utilization of your secondary energy source: fat. You can see why foods that stimulate huge insulin releases may not be the athlete's best friend.

Nutritional scientists have developed the *glycemic index* to help you estimate how much insulin you will produce when you eat a variety of carbohydrates. The higher the value, the faster you'll absorb the carbohydrate. Table 2.2 lists the glycemic index of some of the more common carbohydrates so that you can get to know who your food friends are.

Food	Index	Food	Index
Glucose	100	Banana	60
Cooked carrots	90	Spaghetti	50
Corn flakes	80	All bran	50
Bread	70	Oatmeal	50
White rice	70	Peas	50
Potatoes	70	Apple	40
Raisins	65	Orange	40
Corn	60	Beans	30

Table 2.2. The glycemic index of some common foods.

Your body can store glucose in your liver and muscles by forming long chains of glucose called *glycogen*. The glycogen stored in your liver can be used to maintain a normal blood-sugar level during exercise. Unlike the glycogen stored in your liver, glycogen stored in muscles primarily serves as an energy source for the muscle where it is stored.

Glycogen has an osmotic effect, meaning that it attracts water. It can help you store an extra 1.5 liters of water in your muscles. When you exercise, your muscles will use your glycogen for energy, and the water that's released can help you stay hydrated.

With the glycogen that you have stored in your liver and muscles, you have enough energy to sustain a moderate level of exercise for approximately two to three hours. During the first two hours of exercise, glucose and glycogen will be your main energy source, and the amount of protein and fat that you burn will be small. As you continue to exercise, you'll deplete your glycogen stores and your body will utilize more fat and protein. Although you will be able to continue to exercise with fat as your primary fuel source, you will not be able to perform as well (Fitts 1996).

Not only do your muscles prefer glucose, your brain also requires it as its primary energy source. Once your blood sugar drops, your ability to think and respond appropriately will begin to decline. As a backup measure, your body can respond to glycogen depletion by scavenging protein molecules and converting them into a small amount of glucose. This process is called *gluconeogenesis*, and although it can only produce enough glucose to maintain exercise levels at 40% of your maximum, it is one of the ways that your body maintains adequate glucose levels for your brain during prolonged exercise (Ivy 1999).

Since fat and protein can't provide enough energy to keep you running at your best, you can understand why it is so important to get some carbohydrates during a long event. We'll discuss what type and how much later in this chapter.

Optimal Protein

Proteins are made up of building blocks called *amino acids*. There are twenty-one amino acids, and your body can make eleven of them. The remaining ten are called essential because you need to get them from your diet. The quality of a protein describes how many essential amino acids are present in a given meal. Complete proteins contain all the essential amino acids in relatively high amounts, whereas incomplete proteins are missing one or more of the essential amino acids.

You can get the full spectrum of essential amino acids by combining incomplete protein sources that compliment each other. The good news is you don't need to eat them all in the same meal to get the right combination of amino acids; you have up to twenty-four hours to get the right combination. Examples of incomplete protein sources that complement each other are rice and beans or bread and milk. See Table 2.3 for more complementary protein combinations.

Complementary Proteins

Tofu with veggies and rice	Beans and rice
Peanut butter with bread	Cereal and milk
Cornbread with baked beans	Bread and milk

Table 2.3. Complementary proteins.

Athletes need protein to build stronger muscles. Specialized proteins called *enzymes* facilitate thousands of essential chemical reactions in your body and play a major role in energy production. The amount of protein that you need is a matter of controversy. At the lower end of the spectrum is the RDA at 0.4 grams per pound of lean body weight per day (g/lb/d). For athletes involved in heavy physical training, some sports nutritionists recommend daily protein intakes of 0.5–0.8 g/lb/d (Lemon 1995, 1996; Rankin 1999). See Table 2.4 for more guidelines about protein intake.

Based on these recommendations, a 150-pound athlete will need between 75 and 120 grams of protein per day. During your harder training cycles, you may want to stay closer to the higher number. Assuming that you don't have health problems, protein intake within this range is reasonably safe, and the amino acids that you don't use can be converted into glucose for energy.

If you eat meat and diary products, it will be easy to meet your daily protein needs. Vegetarians can get enough protein by combining the proper food groups.

Some athletes choose to increase their protein intake with protein supplements. Although this isn't necessary, the demands of a hectic training schedule can make it difficult to get enough protein from your food. Athletes who are concerned about the high levels of fat and cholesterol in animal products can also choose protein supplements that are low in fat and cholesterol. In these circumstances, protein supplementation may provide a reasonable alternative for the busy athlete.

Weight in Pounds	Protein Intake in Grams
100	50–80
125	62–100
150	75–120
175	87–140
200	100–160
225	112–180
250	125–200

Table 2.4 Maximal daily protein requirements.

To make things just a little more complicated, protein supplements come in a variety of formulations. Intact proteins from milk, whey, egg, or soy are called *polypeptides* whereas proteins that have been broken down into smaller chains of one, two, or three amino acids are called *hydrolysates*.

Formulations containing individual amino acids or combinations of *free-form amino acids* (including aspartate, arginine, ornithine, lysine, glutamine, and glycine) and *branched chain amino acids* (including tryptophan) are being marketed as performance-enhancing agents. Unfortunately it's hard to find enough scientific evidence to genuinely support these claims (Williams 1999).

If you decide to supplement your protein intake, your best bet is to stick with the polypeptides and hydrolysates. The amino acid combinations in these products typically mirror those found in nature. They are also the least damaging to your pocketbook compared to other protein supplements.

Again, food is the best way to get your protein, and your best bet is to make protein supplementation the exception and not the rule. Refer to Table 2.5 for more protein sources.

Protein Sources	
20 to 30 grams	**5 to 10 grams**
Beef (3 oz.)	Bagel (1)
Chicken breast (3 oz.)	Wheat bread (2 slices)
Tuna (3 oz.)	Cooked beans (1/2 cup)
Turkey (3 oz.)	Nuts (1 oz.)

	Protein Sources
	Rice (1 cup, cooked)
10-20 grams	Spaghetti (1 cup)
Fish (3 oz.)	Yogurt (8 oz.)
Chicken drumstick	Milk (1 cup)
Pork (3 oz.)	Cheese (1 oz.)
Bran muffin	Wheat germ (1 oz.)
Tofu (1/2 cup)	Whole cereals (1 cup)

Table 2.5. Protein content of various foods.

Spare the Fat

It seemed that for some time, fat was the odd man out when it came to athletic performance. Some groups were recommending diets containing 10% of the calories from fat, but recently some authors have recommended fat intakes as high as 30% (Sears). Fat intakes of more than 30% appear to have an adverse effect on performance and health (Tourcotte 1999). The American Heart Association recommends that 20% to 30% of your caloric intake should come from fat, with less than 10% of your calories coming from *saturated fats*.

Just so you don't get mixed up, it's important to note that we're talking about the percentage of calories from fat and not the percentage of fat by weight. For example, 2% low-fat milk is 2% fat by weight but approximately 35% of the calories from low-fat milk come from fat.

Fat is your most concentrated source of energy. It weighs in at 9 calories per gram compared to roughly 3.5 calories per gram for a protein or carbohydrate. One of the reasons that fat is such a concentrated form of energy is that unlike glycogen, your body can store fat without water. As a result, after a couple of hours of exercise you'll have depleted your glycogen stores, but you can still rely on your fat stores to keep you moving for days.

In addition to providing energy, fats perform a variety of important functions in your body:

- Transportation of fat-soluble vitamins
- Providing a structural component for cell membranes and nerve sheaths

- Serving as a precursor to various hormones and hormonelike substances called prostaglandins
- Providing insulation for temperature control and cushioning of vital organs
- Dietary fats also provide taste to your food and contribute to the overall sense of satisfaction from your meal

The fat in your diet is frequently described as saturated, monounsaturated, or polyunsaturated. Due to their solid nature, saturated fats increase your risk for heart disease whereas monounsaturated and polyunsaturated fats are preferred in part because they tend to be liquids and are less likely to become a solid that clogs your arteries. Polyunsaturated fats can also be distinguished by their chemical configuration. Fats that contain omega-3 fatty acids are found in coldwater fish including salmon, mackerel, and sardines, as well as in oils from flax seed or walnuts (Halbert 1997).

Sorting out the dietary sources of saturated and unsaturated fats can be simplified by remembering that most meat, poultry, and dairy fats are relatively high in saturated fats, as are palm and coconut oils (tropical oils). The fats found in fish and vegetable oils are typically unsaturated, whereas safflower, sunflower, and corn oil lead the way in polyunsaturation.

Linoleic acid and linolenic acid are fatty acids that are not manufactured by your body in adequate amounts and hence are considered essential fatty acids. It's important that you get a reasonable amount of these essential fatty acids because you'll need them to make chemicals called prostaglandins. These chemicals have hormonelike effects on your blood vessels and intestines.

The good news is that it is relatively easy to get the proper levels of essential fatty acids in your diet by including corn, safflower, and soybean oils as well as walnuts, sunflower seeds, almonds, and peanut butter.

Hydrogenation is a process that manipulates the saturation of a fatty acid by adding hydrogen to the carbon double bonds of a polyunsaturated fat. An example would be to hydrogenate corn oil to make margarine so that the oil remains solid at room temperature. Making your margarine hard seems like a good idea until you consider that process of hydrogenation will alter certain aspects of the fatty acid molecule that make it less desirable from a nutritional perspective (Halbert, 1997). Furthermore, high levels saturated fat intake may increase your risk of heart disease and certain forms of cancer. You may want to limit your intake of saturated fats to less than 10% of your total caloric intake.

All the Vitamins and Minerals

There is no doubt that your body needs vitamins for optimal growth and performance. Vitamins are complex organic molecules that are typically found in foods. Some important vitamin-dependent processes include bone growth, immunity, energy production, nervous system function, good vision, healthy skin, and normal red blood cell production. Because of the essential role that vitamins play in health and performance, you'll want to be sure to get the right amount from your diet.

There are thirteen vitamins. Vitamins A, D, E, and K are fat soluble, whereas the eight B vitamins and vitamin C are water soluble. You have some flexibility with your day-to-day intake of fat-soluble vitamins because your body can store the fat-soluble vitamins for substantial periods. On the other hand, water-soluble vitamins are rapidly eliminated from your body, so you need to make sure that you get an adequate supply on a regular basis. If your intake of vitamins C, D, or niacin is chronically deficient, you could be at risk of developing diseases like scurvy, rickets, or pellagra. Although the signs of some vitamin deficiencies may take years to develop, it is generally recommended that you get a good supply of water-soluble vitamins on a daily basis.

From the athlete's perspective, disease prevention is not the main concern because most of these diseases are quite rare in developed countries. The main question that athletes have is if there is an optimal level of vitamin intake that maximizes athletic performance.

Fortunately, under most circumstances, you can get all vitamins that you need from a well-balanced diet but it takes some effort. Keep in mind that you can only eat a limited number of calories per day so you'll want to do your best to avoid empty calories. You can increase your chances of getting the right amount of vitamins by eating a variety of nutritious foods from different sources.

The way your food is stored and prepared will also affect its vitamin content. Processing, heating, freezing, canning, and prolonged storage will decrease the vitamin content of most foods as will boiling, frying, or overcooking your food.

Optimally, you should strive to eat foods that are properly cleansed, fresh, and only lightly cooked, if cooking is necessary. Certain foods, primarily meats and eggs, need to be adequately cooked to prevent transmission of bacteria and parasites.

The Recommended Daily Allowance (RDA) for vitamins is set at a point that is above the amount needed to prevent deficiency yet well below the level that causes toxicity. Whether vitamin intakes above the RDA improve health and athletic performance is a matter of controversy with experts and nonexperts lining up on either side of the issue. Very few scientific studies have been able to prove that vitamin supplementation improves health or athletic performance in individuals with good dietary habits. See Table 2.6 for the RDAs for adult males.

Good food is still the best way to get your vitamins, and there are other nutrients in food that you can't replace with pills.

On the other hand, there could be times when you don't have control over the storage and preparation of your food or when good food just isn't available. Under these circumstances you may have trouble getting your basic allowance of vitamins. When you consider the low cost and safety of supplementation at RDA levels, it gets hard to argue against basic supplementation.

Well, if a little is good, can more be better? It's hard to find any convincing evidence that megadoses of vitamins offer you any clear advantage and in some situations they can cause significant toxicity. Your chances of developing toxicity are greatest with the fat-soluble vitamins but that doesn't mean toxicity can't occur with the water-soluble vitamins. You may want to avoid supplementation at high levels without first consulting your family physician.

For athletes, one exception may be vitamin C. Several studies have suggested that supplementation at levels above the RDA may provide protection against respiratory infections in individuals that are under heavy physical stress (Hemila 1996). In addition, vitamin C may exert a protective effect against exercise-induced muscle damage (Jakeman 1993). Doses up to 250 mg a day have been well tolerated in adults. Again, in rare instances toxicity may develop even at these levels, so be sure to contact your family physician prior to supplementation above the RDA level.

Vitamin	Name	RDA	Function	Dietary Source
A	Retinol (Carotene)	900 mcg	Healthy skin, hair, and nails; night vision	Deep yellow or orange fruits and vegetables
D	Cholecalciferol	5 to 10 mcg (AI)	Improves calcium absorption for healthy teeth and bones	Egg yolks, fortified dairy products, fish liver oils, and sunlight

Vitamin	Name	RDA	Function	Dietary Source
E	Tocopherol	15 mg	Antioxidant, preserves fatty acids, and plays role in cell formation	Seeds, nuts, wheat germ, poultry, seafood, and eggs.
K		120 mcg (AI)	Blood clotting and bone health	Green, leafy vegetables; whole grains; potatoes; cabbage. Your intestinal bacteria also produce Vitamin K.
C	Ascorbic Acid	90 mg	Antioxidant; cellular health and immunity	Fresh fruit (especially citrus); fresh vegetables including cauliflower, broccoli, and peppers.
B1	Thiamine	1.2 mg	Carbohydrate metabolism; nerve and digestive function	Grains, seafood, veggies
B2	Riboflavin	1.3 mg	Food metabolism and energy production	Meats, dairy, and grains; dark green, leafy vegetables
B3	Niacin (Nicotinic Acid)	16 mg	Energy metabolism, growth, and digestion	Seafood, nuts, whole grains
B5	Pantothenic Acid	5 mg (AI)	Food metabolism	Eggs, nuts, grains, meats; also produced by your intestinal bacteria
B6	Pyridoxine	1.3 mg	Protein and carbohydrate metabolism, nerve function	Meats, whole grains, potatoes, bananas
B12	Cobalamin	2.4 mcg	Red cell production, nerve function	Meat and dairy products
Folic Acid	Folate	400 mcg	Red cell production, genetic material	Fruits, vegetables, legumes, whole grains

Vitamin	Name	RDA	Function	Dietary Source
Biotin		30 mcg (AI)	Food metabolism	Meats, legumes, and vegetables; also produced by your intestinal bacteria.

Table 2.6. Vitamins. (Amounts are for adult males unless specified. AI-adequate intake where there is no RDA established. See USDA website for detailed information: http://www.nal.usda.gov/fnic/etext/000105.html)

Know Which Foods are Rich in the Minerals

Unlike vitamins, minerals are basic elements that exist as ionic salts. They are called ionic salts because they carry a small electric charge and therefore need to combine with an oppositely charged molecule to form a salt. That's why the contents of your mineral supplements are expressed as ferrous sulfate or magnesium oxide.

Minerals work together with other molecules in your body to perform a variety of important functions. For example, calcium plays an important role in the structure of your bones and in the normal functioning of your muscles, whereas iron is the central component of the hemoglobin molecule. There are thirteen essential minerals, and they have been listed along with their primary functions and dietary sources in Table 2.7.

Under most circumstances, you'll be able to get all the minerals you need from a healthy diet. One problem that may affect the mineral content of your food is the quality of the soil where your food is grown. In many parts our country, the soils have become depleted of minerals, however, with the use of chemical fertilizers our farmers are able to produce healthy-looking fruits, vegetables, and grains that may be lacking in essential minerals. In most urban areas it's difficult to determine the source of your food and, hence, the mineral content. If you have a choice, you may want to consider getting your foods from a variety of geographic areas and from suppliers that attend to proper soil maintenance.

The good news is that trace minerals are needed in very tiny amounts, and your body is able to store them for a substantial length of time. Notwithstanding the above, athletes need to be sure that they are consistently getting an adequate level of minerals. Let's take a look at the minerals that your body needs.

Minerals			
Name	**RDA***	**Function**	**Dietary sources**
Calcium	1000–1300 mg	Bone strength, muscle, and nerve function	Milk products, tofu, and dark green, leafy vegetables
Phosphorous	700 mg	Bone strength, nerve, and muscle function, energy chain, pH balance	Dairy, meats, peas
Magnesium	♂420 mg ♀320 mg	Enzyme cofactor in a variety of biological systems	Beans and nuts, Green, leafy veggies, whole grain cereals and bread
Iron	♂8mg ♀18 mg	Oxygen transport	Meat and poultry, cast-iron pots, and fortified grains.
Zinc	♂11 mg ♀8 mg	Cofactor in energy production, metabolism, and testosterone production	Oysters, beef, whole grains, and wheat germ
Copper	900 mcg	Iron utilization, enzyme cofactor	Organ meats, nuts, whole grains, and seafood
Selenium	55 mcg	Antioxidant	Seafood, whole grains, eggs, and garlic
Chromium	35mcg(AI)	Works with insulin	Whole grains, nuts, and brewer's yeast
Iodine	150 mcg	Thyroid function	Seafood, iodized salt, vegetables from iodine-rich soils
Fluoride	4 mg (AI)	Prevents tooth decay	Fluoridated water
Manganese	2.3 mg (AI)	Enzyme cofactor; tendon and bone structure	Tea, nuts, beans, and whole grains
Molybdenum		Enzyme cofactor	Green, leafy vegetables
Sulfur		Amino acid component	Wheat germ, beans, and beef

Table 2.7. Minerals. Amounts are for adult males unless specified. AI-adequate intake where there is no RDA established. See USDA website for detailed information: http://www.nal.usda.gov/fnic/etext/000105.html

Mineral deficiencies affect athletic performance in several common scenarios. The first is when iron deficiency affects endurance athletes and female athletes. It's not surprising that some athletes get low on iron because your gastrointestinal tract has a limited ability to absorb iron, and endurance athletes have been known to lose iron through their sweat, their gastrointestinal tract, and their urinary tract. In addition, female athletes lose iron during their menstrual cycles. If your intake can't keep up with your losses, you'll soon become deficient.

During the early stages of iron depletion, you'll notice little, if any, effect on performance, but once you become anemic you'll see a marked decrease in energy and performance.

Before you run off and add carpentry nails to your breakfast, the truth is that most athletes won't need iron supplementation as long as they eat enough iron-rich foods. In addition, some individuals have difficulty tolerating large amounts of iron, and in normal individuals excess iron has no special performance-enhancing effects. To complicate matters, iron deficiency may develop because of an under-lying disease and taking iron to treat the low red blood cell concentration that characterizes anemia may only delay the diagnosis. If you suspect that you are at risk for iron deficiency, your best bet is to see your doctor.

Getting enough calcium is a special concern for female athletes because calcium plays an important role in maximizing bone strength. We'll talk about the relationship between estrogen, calcium, vitamin D, and bone density in another section, but let me just say for now that calcium and vitamin D play a critical role in bone growth and maintenance.

Dairy products are a good source of calcium, and although you can get some calcium from figs, apricots, tofu, beans, greens, and kelp, you'll have to eat bucketfuls to meet your requirements. If you can't tolerate dairy products, your best bet is to talk to your doctor about lactose intolerance or consider taking an appropriate calcium supplement. To get the most out of your calcium intake, you'll need adequate amounts of vitamin D. With fifteen minutes of sunshine a day, your skin can make enough Vitamin D to meet your needs. Food sources include fortified milk, fish liver oils, and egg yolks.

Your body needs phosphorous for a variety of exercise-related functions. Although phosphate deficiency is rare, several studies have suggested that phosphate may improve aerobic performance (Clarkson 1994). Dietary sources of phosphorous include dairy products, eggs, meat, fish, and legumes. Taking excess phosphate may adversely affect your calcium balance, and the safety of loading up on phosphate as a performance-enhancing strategy has yet to be established.

Magnesium is a cofactor in over 325 enzymatic reactions, many of which involve energy production. Magnesium deficiency may reduce physical performance and heavy exercise can lead to magnesium depletion (Bohl 2002). Adequate magnesium intake may decrease migraines (Holroyd 2003) and muscle cramping (Clarkson 1994). Dietary sources of magnesium include tofu; green leafy vegetables; beans; nuts; fortified, whole grain cereals and breads; oysters; and scallops.

Zinc supplements have been frequently used by athletes, but there is little evidence that supplementation improves athletic performance. Moreover, zinc intake above 50 mg per day may adversely affect copper metabolism. Dietary sources of zinc include beef, oysters, yogurt, fortified cereals, and wheat germ.

Various sports magazines promote chromium supplementation as an ergogenic or performance-enhancing aid and fat burner. Unfortunately, well-controlled studies have been unable to demonstrate significant strength gains, increased lean body mass, or improved performance with chromium supplementation. In addition, there may be adverse effects related to excess chromium intake (Stearns 1995).

Overall, the evidence for performance enhancement from high amounts of mineral supplementation is limited. There is no strong evidence to support supplementation at levels above the RDA unless it is to treat a specific disorder under the supervision of a physician. If you aren't sure whether you're getting all the minerals that you need from your diet, then taking a mineral supplement at RDA levels might be a good idea. Otherwise, as with vitamins, your best bet is to consume a variety of nutritious foods on a regular basis and avoid the empty calories and nutritional zeros.

Water

You can go weeks without food, months before developing significant vitamin or mineral deficiencies, but without water you'll be in deep trouble after just a couple of days. Water is by far the most essential nutrient. The human body is made up of approximately 60% water and without it you will have difficulty regulating your temperature, maintaining blood pressure, and eliminating waste products.

It's no surprise that you'll need more water during exercise because heavy exertion increases the demands on your circulatory system as well as your cooling system. Losing even 2 % of your body weight to dehydration not only decreases your physical and mental performance, it will significantly impair your ability to tolerate heat. If you let yourself become severely dehydrated, your safety will be compromised (Latzka 1999).

In spite of the importance of staying hydrated, some athletes don't even think about drinking until they become thirsty. With so many factors to attend to during practice and competition, hydration is commonly ignored. This is because your thirst mechanism doesn't kick in until you've lost a substantial amount of water. By the time you get thirsty, you've already lost enough fluid to adversely affect your performance. At that point, it will be difficult to compete while drinking the amount of fluid that you will need to maintain optimal hydration. Since your thirst mechanism is not a good indicator of early dehydration, you'll want to anticipate your fluid needs by drinking before you get thirsty.

Let's start by looking at your basic fluid requirements. If you are just hanging around in cool weather, your fluid requirements are only between 1,000 and 1,500 ml per day. That's about six, eight-ounce glasses of water per day. On the other hand, during a tough workout on a hot day, your fluid losses can be as high as 3,000 ml per *hour*.

The first step to maintaining optimal hydration is to start your workouts fully hydrated by simply drinking water or beverages that contain water. You'll want to avoid beverages that have alcohol or caffeine because they'll increase urine production and eventually you'll lose more fluid than you consume.

At the other end of the spectrum, over-hydrating before competition will increase urine production and unless your sport allows you to run back and forth to the bathroom you'll want to closely monitor your fluid intake. A practical recommendation is to drink 400 to 600 ml of fluid two hours before exercise and 200 to 300 ml immediately before exercise (Latzka 1999).

Drinking too much fluid during exercise can cause bloating and as you start to drink large amounts of water without balanced electrolytes, you can develop electrolyte disturbances that include low sodium and potassium. Using a sport drink can help, but even with electrolyte replacement you need to be aware of the potential of over-hydration and electrolyte problems during events lasting more than four hours or when your fluid intake approaches three liters (Almond et al. 2005).

You can avoid bloating, over-hydration, and electrolyte problems by monitoring the type of fluid that you drink as well as the amount and its temperature. During moderate exercise, most healthy, well-conditioned adult athletes are able to tolerate between 600 and 1000 ml per hour without getting bloated. If you plan to exercise more than one hour, you'll want to consider replacing glucose and electrolytes. Fluids that contain high amounts of sugar will decrease absorption and increase the likelihood of bloating. The optimal glucose concentration to improve performance and limit bloating is between 5% and 8% glucose. As an added benefit, drinking a carbohydrate beverage during prolonged exercise may help your immune system fight off infections (Nieman 1999).

The temperature of the fluid you drink will also affect the rate of absorption. By using a fluid that is approximately 60°F or 70°F you'll improve absorption and maximize the cooling effects on your body (ACSM 1996).

There are a variety of ways to monitor your level of hydration. You can simply make sure that you are producing enough saliva and perspiration as well as an adequate amount of clear urine. To get a more precise estimate of your fluid needs, see Table 2.8. You'll want to weigh yourself before and after exercise, and then measure the amount of fluid that you drank during the workout. The total amount of fluid that you'll need to stay fully hydrated during a similar workout is the sum of the fluid you drank and the weight that you lost (water weighs approximately two pounds per quart). The goal is to drink enough fluid to limit your weight loss to less than 2% of your total body weight. At the same time, you'll want to avoid over-hydrating to a level that would result in weight gain.

Calculating Fluid Losses

pre-exercise weight
- your weight after exercise
= fluid deficit (One pound = 16 oz.)

fluid deficit
+ the amount of fluid taken during exercise
= total fluid needed for a similar workout

Table 2.8. Fluid replacement.

Once you've estimated the amount of fluid that you need for a workout, you can place it in a water bottle and plan to gradually drink the entire bottle over the duration of your workout. For example, if you're planning to drink a quart of fluid during your hour-long workout, try to spread it out by drinking eight ounces every fifteen minutes. The idea is to avoid getting bloated by sipping small amounts as frequently as you can (AFP-ACSM 2006).

Staying optimally hydrated during practice can help you get the most out of your workouts as you get used to drinking the right amount of fluid. You may also want to try a variety of sports drinks during practice so you can decide which one to use during competition.

What you eat before, during, and after exercise will have a substantial effect on your performance and recovery time. Ideally, you're going to want to develop an eating program that is compatible with your training program. By practicing your eating routines along with your workouts, you'll get a better idea of what foods work best for you. Hopefully, you won't make the mistake of experimenting with something new on the day of an important event because if it doesn't agree with you, it will ruin your day.

A good, general recommendation is to begin eating four hours before your workout by consuming 2 grams of carbohydrate per pound of body weight. One hour before your workout, you'll want to get another 0.5 grams of carbohydrate per pound of body weight. (Sherman 1989). You can look at your food labels to find out how much carbohydrate you get from each food. For example, if you weigh 150 pounds, you might have the meal in Table 2.9 four hours prior to competition, followed by a snack one hour before competing.

You may also want to consider trying several pregame eating routines in case one of your basic foods is not available on the big day. I've summarized the carbohydrate content of some common foods in Table 2.10.

Four Hours Before Competition	
Grape-Nuts, 1 cup	100g
Yogurt w/ fruit, 1 cup	50g
2% Milk, 8 oz.	15g
Banana	25g
Apple	20g
Raisins, 1/3 cup	40g
Toast, 2	25g
Jam	15g
Total carbohydrates	**280g**

One Hour Before Competition	
Bagel	30g
Fig Newton	11g
Banana	20g
Sports drink 8 oz.	<u>14g</u>
Total carbohydrates	75g

Table 2.9. Pregame meal.

Food	Carbohydrates	Food	Carbohydrates
Apple	20g	Cooked spaghetti, 1 cup	40g
Banana	25g	Bagel	30g
Orange	15g	Oatmeal cookie	10g
Fig	12g	Cooked brown rice, 1 cup	45g
Raisins, 1.5 oz.	35g	Cooked pinto beans, 1 cup	45g
Bread, 1 slice	12g	Meats, poultry, fish	0
Potato	35g	Milk, 8 oz.	15g
4-inch Pancake	10g	Yogurt w/ fruit, 1 cup	50g

Table 2.10. Carbohydrate content of various foods.

If you're going to be exercising for over an hour, you'll want to consume additional carbohydrates during your workout. You'll maximize your endurance performance by eating or drinking another 0.5 grams of carbohydrate per pound of body weight every hour. You can use your favorite sports bar or try a small amount of dried fruit, bananas, or a bagel. You can improve absorption and avoid excess insulin production by drinking plenty of fluid and avoiding foods with a high glycemic index.

Get Your Diet Together

Now that you have all this information, how are you going to get all the right nutrients into your body? You can always carry around a small computer to measure the exact nutritional content of your food. Another option is to consume a variety of chemically engineered, predigested powders, shakes, and bars in conjunction with several handfuls of pills. This tasteless option is very expensive and offers no significant advantage, not to mention the amount of indigestion you'll experience. Your goal is to consume a diet that satisfies your taste buds, provides you with an optimal level of nutrition, and doesn't wreak havoc with your digestive system.

The first order of business is to maintain adequate caloric balance because a negative caloric balance will make you feel tired and force your body to break down your muscles for energy (Grandjean 1999). Depending on your training load, you may need to chow down anywhere between 1,800 and 6,000 calories a day just to keep up. This can be quite a challenge for the busy, tired athlete who can't afford to be working out with a full stomach. If you want to be at your best, you'll need to have a plan.

One way to keep your caloric intake in balance is to plan three reasonable meals with a couple of healthy snacks every day. You can supplement your caloric intake by using a carbohydrate replacement drink while you train, and you can eat bananas, dried fruit, or a sports bar during your long workouts.

During heavy training cycles you will need to vary the relative amounts of carbohydrate, protein, and fat so that you can get the right amount of calories and macronutrients. It's become popular to discuss macronutrient intake in terms of percentages, but the concept of adhering to a strict percentage has some problems when you have a high-caloric demand (Cheuvront 1999). For example, trying to get 30% of your calories from protein when you need to eat 5,000 calories means that you need 1,500 calories of protein or 440 grams of protein. Even if you weigh 300 pounds, your maximal recommended protein intake would only be 240 grams (0.8 g/pound of body weight).

A better approach is to get the right amount of protein for your body weight first, and then satisfy the rest of your caloric needs with carbohydrates and fat. Since fat is such a concentrated energy source, it would be reasonable to increase your fat intake to 30% during heavy training cycles as long as you stick with healthy, unsaturated fats. Reasonable macronutrient intake can vary between the following ranges depending on your training load:

Carbohydrate	40%–70%
Protein	15%–30%
Fat	15%–30%

While the experts argue about the optimal macronutrient levels, you're going to need to make some decisions about what to eat. It's difficult to calculate the exact intake of each macronutrient, so every day becomes an exercise in estimation.

Even the best estimators are going to be 10% to 15% off, not to mention the effects of day-to-day variability in food intake.

Your best bet is to develop a variety of smart eating routines that you can use whether you're at home or on the run. Once you've established a good base of nutritious food options, you can begin to add and substitute foods so that you don't end up with a boring diet. Eating a variety of foods also improves your chances of getting the entire spectrum of nutrients.

Remember that you can only consume a limited number of calories per day, and they need to be packed with nutrients. Otherwise, you'll never meet your requirements. When you're planning a meal, try to estimate the amount of carbohydrate, protein, and fat in that meal. Once you've estimated the macronutrient content, you can evaluate your meal from the perspective of vitamin and mineral content. I've also added some guidelines to help you identify foods that are high in vitamin and mineral content as well as those foods that are essentially empty calories. Table 2.11 lists good food choices.

Preferred Foods	Avoid
Fresh fruits and veggies	Fried and overcooked foods
Whole grains and legumes	Processed and canned foods
Low fat dairy products	Candies and chips
Lean meats, poultry, & fish	High-fat meat and dairy
Tofu, yogurt	Butter, creams, ice cream
Smoothies, juices	Sodas
Polyunsaturated fats/oils	Saturated fats/oils

Table 2.11. Food choices.

The USDA makes the following recommendations for a 2,000-calorie diet:

- Consume a sufficient amount of fruits and vegetables while staying within energy needs. Two cups of fruit and two and a half cups of vegetables per day are recommended for a 2,000-calorie intake, with higher or lower amounts depending on the calorie level.
- Choose a variety of fruits and vegetables each day. In particular, select from all five vegetable subgroups (dark green, orange, legumes, starchy vegetables, and other vegetables) several times a week.

- Consume three or more ounce-equivalents of whole grain products per day, with the rest of the recommended grains coming from enriched or whole grain products. In general, at least half the grains should come from whole grains.
- Consume three cups per day of fat-free or low-fat milk or equivalent milk products (USDA 2005).

Our bodies are designed to absorb nutrients in the natural forms and combinations found in food. When properly prepared and presented, food not only provides the best in nutritional value, it is also very enjoyable and satisfying to eat. As a tired, hungry athlete, you'll want to take advantage of the opportunity to recover by sitting down and having a healthy meal with a friend.

Chapter 3

Get in Shape

Running out of gas before the game is over? Having trouble keeping up? Maybe it's time to get in better shape. From the athletic perspective, being fit means that you'll be able to endure high intensity exercise longer than your competitor. On the health side, you'll have a lower risk for heart disease, lower blood pressure, stronger bones, and lower body fat. Regardless of your sport, you can reap the benefits of better health and performance by improving your level of aerobic conditioning. In this chapter we will review some of the basic concepts related to cardiovascular fitness as well as some of the practical methods of improving speed, endurance, and recovery.

Basic Physiology

One of the critical factors in any form of sustained exercise is your ability to deliver oxygen to your muscles. We'll need to review some basic biochemistry to help you understand how you produce energy from food and oxygen. In the previous chapter, we learned that glucose is the primary fuel source for exercise, but before you can use it, your body has to break it down. The process of breaking down glucose is called *glycolysis* as illustrated in Table 3.1. During glycolysis, glucose is converted into a small amount of energy and an important molecule called *pyruvate*. The fate of pyruvate depends on how much oxygen you have available in your muscles. Under **aerobic** conditions, plenty of oxygen exists and the continued breakdown of pyruvate yields a substantial amount of *ATP* (adenosine triphosphate). ATP is important because it is the main energy source for muscle contraction during prolonged exercise.

Under *anaerobic* conditions, the lack of oxygen blocks the production of ATP and pyruvate is converted to **lactic acid**. As lactic acid accumulates in your muscles, you will begin to experience pain and fatigue and eventually will have to slow down or stop. The big difference between aerobic and anaerobic exercise is that under aerobic conditions, the breakdown of glucose yields nineteen times more energy in the form of ATP than under anaerobic conditions (Table 3.1 Glycolysis). Because your cardiovascular and pulmonary systems are responsible for oxygen delivery, you're going to want to know how to maximize their performance.

If you have to pace yourself during a long event or endurance competition, you'll need to keep in mind that pushing yourself into the anaerobic zone means you'll use up your glycogen stores at a faster rate.

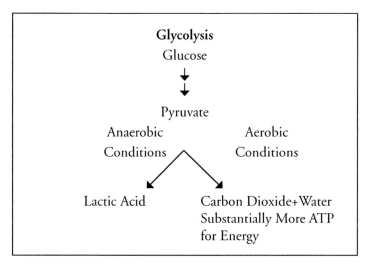

Table 3.1. Glycolysis.

Your body can utilize a variety of energy sources depending on the intensity and duration of your activity. For very short, high intensity activities like the shot put, single jump, or single weight lifting events, your muscles look to stored ATP and creatine phosphate for energy. If your sport requires repetitive bouts of short, high intensity activities, then you can optimize performance by maintaining adequate creatine stores though dietary sources like meats and fish or through supplementation (Stricker 1998). When you need energy for longer, high intensity anaerobic activities such as sprints, your muscles will begin the process of glycolysis to turn glycogen into ATP and lactic acid. Finally, with lower intensity aerobic activities, your muscles will use glycolysis in combination with aerobic metabolism to convert glycogen into ATP.

We've been talking about your muscles in a general sense, but in reality, you have three types of specialized skeletal muscle fibers, each of which is adapted for different types of activity. Type I fibers are commonly called *slow twitch fibers* because they are rich in glycogen and well suited for endurance activities within the aerobic range. An example of a Type I activity would be long-distance running. Type IIa fibers are *fast twitch fibers* that also utilize glucose and glycogen but primarily for glycolysis and anaerobic metabolism. They're specifically adapted for activities that require a short burst of speed, such as sprinting, and can handle substantially higher levels of lactic acid. Type IIb fibers are *fast twitch fibers,* and they are rich in ATP and creatine phosphate. They perform best in very short, high intensity activities such as throwing a shot put.

Every person has a different amount of each muscle fiber type, and the percentages that you have are determined by your genetic makeup. In spite of your genetic predisposition, you can manipulate how your type IIa fibers behave by the type of training you do. Endurance training will modify some Type IIa fibers so that they behave like Type I fibers. Alternatively, explosive, high intensity training will make Type IIa fibers behave like IIb fibers. Type I and Type IIb fibers don't change very much (Cahill 1997).

Now that you have an understanding of the basics, let's walk you through a workout from start to finish. At rest, your muscles have adequate stores of oxygen, ATP, and glucose. With the onset of activity, the ATP/creatine phosphate stores in your IIb fibers will carry you through the initial seconds of motion. As you continue to exercise you'll exhaust your ATP stores and your IIb fibers will begin to fatigue. That's when you begin to rely on IIa fibers and glycolysis. This will carry you over until you begin to accumulate lactic acid. It's the level of acidity in your blood that increases your respiratory rate and heart rate, allowing you to maintain normal oxygen levels for your endurance fibers. In the long run, it's your Type I fibers that keep you moving.

The abrupt decrease in oxygen level at the start of exercise is frequently called *oxygen debt.* During low intensity exercise, your cardiovascular system is able to provide enough oxygen to maintain aerobic metabolism and pay off the oxygen debt that you accumulated at the start of exercise. Once your cardiovascular system has adapted to a steady level of exercise, your respiratory rate and heart rate will actually stabilize, and as long as you maintain the same intensity of exercise, your body should operate at a relatively steady state until you run out of fuel.

If you increase your exercise intensity, you will increase your oxygen demand, and your body will go through another adjustment. As long as your cardiovascular system can deliver enough oxygen, you'll maintain aerobic metabolism, and you'll be able to continue exercising at the same intensity for a relatively long time.

At some point, if you continue to increase your exercise intensity, you will eventually outpace your ability to deliver oxygen, and you'll start to produce higher levels of lactic acid. This transition from aerobic metabolism to anaerobic metabolism is referred to as the *anaerobic threshold*. From a functional perspective you can define the anaerobic threshold as the maximal exercise intensity that you can maintain for fifty minutes (Loat 1993). This is an important concept because your anaerobic threshold is a good indicator of your level of aerobic conditioning.

If you continue to exercise above your anaerobic threshold, you'll exceed your ability to deliver oxygen and lactic acid levels will rise to the point where you just can't go anymore. The point at which you've reached your maximal exercise capacity can be measured in terms of the maximal amount of oxygen that you can consume and is called your *maximal oxygen consumption* (*VO2max*). This point is an indicator of your level of fitness, and to some degree, of your aerobic potential. You can measure your VO2max directly using sophisticated equipment or it can be estimated based on your performance during treadmill testing.

The recovery process begins once you return to your baseline level of activity. If you are in good shape, you'll quickly pay back any remaining oxygen debt, and you'll be ready for the next challenge.

If you're not in shape, you're going to hate it.

With the right amount of training, your body will make dramatic adaptations that will maximize your aerobic performance. Within weeks you'll improve both the delivery and utilization of oxygen by your circulatory, respiratory, and musculoskeletal systems. Your heart will be able to pump more blood with each beat because the challenges of aerobic activity will make your heart bigger and stronger. Stronger respiratory muscles will make it easier for you to breathe. Finally, at the muscular level, you'll see more capillaries as well as more mitochondria, the specialized structures in your cells that make ATP.

You will see improvements in your maximal oxygen consumption during the first few months of working out, but most fully grown athletes will stop improving after several months of intense aerobic conditioning. At this point, you've reached your genetic ceiling for maximal oxygen consumption. If your sport requires a high level of aerobic performance you may want to measure your VO2max. These sports include cycling, swimming, running, cross-country skiing, and other sports that require prolonged, high-level exertion.

Have What It Takes

If you are aspiring to become a champion of the *Tour de France*, you will be competing against cyclists with some of the best genetic potentials for aerobic performance. If your VO2max is substantially lower, you're going to have a difficult time keeping up with the competition during repeated aerobic challenges. Granted, there are other factors that affect performance in bicycle racing, but VO2max is one of the most important. Before you invest a great deal of time and money pursuing a sport that requires a high degree of aerobic power, you may want to compare your maximal oxygen consumption to athletes that are competing successfully in your sport. If your VO2max is within the same general range as other athletes that compete at that level, you've got a shot at staying in the pack. If not, you're going to suffer.

Keep in mind that although VO2max is an important predictor of performance in aerobic events, other factors can affect your overall success. These include efficiency of motion, endurance, pacing, and anaerobic threshold. In sports such as swimming and cross county skiing, efficiency and technique have a major effect on performance. Even though these sports require a high level of aerobic ability, it would not be surprising to see a technically skilled athlete beat out a genetically gifted competitor. For example, intermediate level swimmers may get more out of improving their technique than by working on speed and endurance (O'Toole 1995).

Even though your maximal oxygen consumption will not increase after several months of hard training, your ability to perform high intensity aerobic activity may continue to improve because of improved efficiency of motion as well as other adaptations that increase your anaerobic threshold. These adaptations can result in improved aerobic performance over months and possibly years of training. Figure 3.2 illustrates the relationship between VO2max, anaerobic threshold, and duration of training.

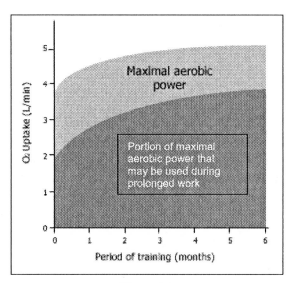

Figure3.2
The relationship between maximal oxygen consumption and anaerobic threshold.

Understand the Aerobic Demands of Your Sport

Most sports can be divided into three main categories based on their aerobic requirements. Activities that are primarily aerobic place minimal demands above the anaerobic threshold and can be further divided into low, medium, and high intensity. Sports that require both sustained aerobic activity with frequent excursions above your anaerobic threshold are referred to as *mixed*. Finally, sports that require primarily short, high intensity activities are considered to be anaerobic. Table 3.2 outlines which sports fall under each category.

Aerobic	Mixed		Anaerobic	
Long Distance:			Sprints while:	
Running	Skiing	Volleyball	Running	Throwing
Swimming	Surfing	Tennis	Swimming	Shot put
Cycling	Basketball	Racquetball	Cycling	Power lifting
Cross-country skiing	Football	Wrestling	Rowing	Single jumps
Walking	Soccer	Jiu-jitsu		
Rowing	Water polo	Karate		

Table 3.2. The aerobic characteristics of various sports.

If you are in a sport that requires intense aerobic demands, then improving your level of aerobic fitness will allow you to perform at a higher level for a longer time. In addition, the physiological stress of high intensity activity will diminish as your level of aerobic fitness improves. You can see why it's important to be fit if you are involved in sport that is aerobically demanding because your ability to develop good skills depends on the amount of high intensity practice you can perform. If you're physiologically stressed by the aerobic challenge, then not only will your high intensity practice time get limited, it will also take you longer to recover for your next workout.

How can you improve your aerobic performance? Let's take a look at how pacing, interval training, and endurance training can keep you at the front of the pack.

Pace Yourself

You need to be able to monitor your level of exertion to keep from running out of gas before the end of the event. You'll develop most of your pacing skills through experience, but you can also monitor your heart rate to get some objective feedback of how hard you are working. If you are generally healthy, your heart rate will be a good indicator of your level of exertion.

Since a major part of pacing is trying to get the feel for when you are reaching your anaerobic threshold, you'll want to know what your heart rate is when you're approaching your anaerobic threshold. Your sports medicine physician can help you determine your heart rate at your anaerobic threshold by monitoring it at various exercise intensities using a treadmill or exercise bicycle. The challenge is to gradually increase your exercise intensity until you reach the highest level that you can sustain for fifty minutes. The key word here is sustainable because by definition it is difficult to sustain intensities above your anaerobic threshold for fifty minutes. Since your heart rate is relatively stable at this level of exertion, it shouldn't be too difficult to determine your heart rate at your anaerobic threshold.

By determining this number, you can monitor your heart rate during exercise and use the information as an objective indicator of your workload. The amount of work that you can do at your anaerobic threshold is also a good indicator of your level of aerobic fitness (Boulay 1997). For example, if you were to test yourself on treadmill at the beginning of your training program, you might notice that the highest speed that you can maintain for fifty minutes is six miles per hour and that your heart rate is cruising at 170 beats per minute. Increasing the pace is uncomfortable and your heart rate will shoot up above your steady rate. Now that you've determined your heart rate at your anaerobic threshold, you can monitor your heart rate during exercise and know that as you approach 170 beats per minute, that you are not going to be able to go much harder without having to back off.

As you continue to train you'll be in better shape, and if you repeat the test you might find that you can sustain a pace of eight miles per hour at a heart rate of 170. The fact that you can sustain higher workload is a good indicator that your hard work has paid off in the form of improved aerobic conditioning. You can monitor your workload at your anaerobic threshold several times throughout the year as a way of keeping track of your level of aerobic fitness.

You can monitor your heart rate by trying to count your pulse occasionally. But if you are serious, you'll want to get an electronic heart rate monitor. Even the basic models are programmable and can be set to beep when you are outside of your desired training range. Some heart rate monitors can store the information from a training session so that you can get feedback regarding the amount of time you spent below, within, and above your target range.

Using your heart rate monitor to measure your exercise intensity is a good way to set your weekly training goals. By using a continuous heart rate monitor, you can set specific goals for your workout intensity and get objective feedback on how well you are meeting those goals.

A heart rate monitor can also help you improve your pacing during competition. Let's take a 10 kilometer race to illustrate how monitoring your heart rate can improve your performance. At the start of the race, everyone is excited and full of energy. The tendency is to get off to a faster pace than you can normally sustain and then get a rude awakening at the half-mile mark. By the time you start to get back to your racing pace, you typically get to the first hill and there's no way you're going to let that overweight, middle-aged runner that just passed you beat you to the top of the hill. You pour it on only to find that there's a fire in each of your legs and that it's probably going to take the rest of the race to put it out.

Had you monitored your heart rate, you could have had immediate feedback that you were going at an unsustainable pace. Experienced athletes learn how to maintain an optimal pace by developing a good sense of their highest sustainable intensity. Using a continuous heart rate monitor can give you important feedback to help you develop this sense.

Interval Training

One way to improve your aerobic performance is to do interval training. This technique involves short intervals of exercise above your anaerobic threshold separated by an active recovery during which you maintain low to medium level of intensity. By pushing yourself above your anaerobic threshold, you gently challenge your cardiovascular and musculoskeletal systems to perform at higher levels.

Once you know your heart rate at your anaerobic threshold, you can use this information to monitor your intensity during interval training. By monitoring your heart rate during recovery, you'll know when you've recovered enough for the next interval. Interval training isn't just valuable for aerobic sports. Athletes that are involved in high intensity anaerobic activities can also benefit from aerobic interval training (Gaiga 1995). Check out Figure 3.4 for an example of a basic interval workout for an athlete with an anaerobic threshold at a heart rate of 165 beats per minute.

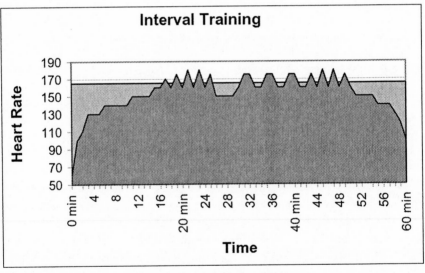

Figure 3.4. Interval training.

Depending on your needs, you can structure your interval workouts in a way that results in either improved aerobic performance or increased speed. Maintaining a lower intensity with shorter rest periods will lead to improved aerobic performance, whereas higher intensity challenges with longer rest periods will increase speed.

Improve your Stamina

No matter how talented you are, if you can't get to the other side of the court in the final period of competition, you're going to be in trouble. That's why if your sport involves long periods of training and competition, you'll want to develop an effective endurance program. The way to improve your endurance is by performing progressively longer, low intensity workouts separated by adequate recovery periods. In addition to improving your cardiovascular fitness, endurance workouts will get your musculoskeletal system ready for prolonged physical challenges.

You can get the most out of your endurance training by monitoring your heart rate and keeping it below your anaerobic threshold. Once you've developed a sense for your endurance-training pace, you can begin to focus on your overall training load. To minimize your risk of injury, you'll want to gradually increase your training time by 10% a week.

Cross-training has become popular among many athletes because it offers a variety of ways to improve endurance and cardiovascular fitness without the repetitive trauma and boredom of participating in just one activity. Cross-training also offers the advantage of improving strength and endurance in a variety of muscle groups whereas participating in a single activity such as running may result in muscle imbalances. You can also incorporate traditional resistance training as part of your cross-training program to improve your running and cycling performance (Tanaka 1998).

The concept of developing strength and endurance throughout your body is important because weakness in one muscle group will decrease your efficiency while increasing the workload on other muscle groups. For example, tennis players with weak abdominal muscles will place increased pressure on their upper extremities during repetitive serving and overhead volleys. You can avoid straining and subsequently weakening a muscle group by developing a well-rounded fitness program. The added benefit of becoming familiar with a variety of workout routines will also give you a head start on your recovery when an injury occurs.

Some of the benefits of cross-training within similar muscle groups can be carried over to activities involving the same muscle groups. For example, training on a stair-stepping machine can improve your running performance if you are not a trained runner. As you get to higher levels of performance, *specificity* becomes more critical. That is to say, if you want to improve your 10-K racing time, your best bet is to spend plenty of time running at your desired 10-K racing pace. As you get closer to your event, you can add some shorter, high intensity workouts.

Specificity also applies to the muscle groups you are training as well as how you are training them. This means that although swimming may improve your cardiovascular fitness; don't expect any miraculous improvements in your running performance. Furthermore, the intensity of your training is also quite specific, so if your sport requires anaerobic activities, then you'll need to train those muscle groups with high intensity challenges. These activities include resistance training, plyometrics, and sprints. Resistance training involves shortening a muscle from a fixed position. Plyometrics are exercises that typically load and lengthen a muscle before the direction of contraction changes. An example of plyometric exercise is having to jump from a fixed position and then having to jump immediately after landing. Sprints are exercises that require a burst of speed for a short period of time. We'll discuss these three types of activities more in the next chapter.

High Altitude Training

Some athletes believe that training at high altitude may have a valuable effect on their level of performance at sea level. Unfortunately, while training at high altitude can have a beneficial effect on your high altitude performance, it probably has minimal if any effect on your performance at sea level. There may be some evidence that living at high altitude while training at sea level improves aerobic performance at sea level, but this remains controversial because the improvement may be subtle and can be outweighed by the amount of time and energy needed to move back and forth from one altitude to the other. This approach also may be more hassle than it's worth.

Getting Your Aerobic Training Program Together: Periodization

The intensity and focus of your training program should vary throughout the year. Typically, you'll want to be at your peak level of conditioning for only certain parts of the year. This is because the level of training that results in peak conditioning can only be maintained for a short period of time before you begin to show signs of fatigue, overtraining, and injury.

The concept of *periodization* prepares the athlete for intense training and competition by breaking the year down to various stages of training. These different stages include:

- Periods of relative rest
- Aerobic conditioning
- Strengthening
- Practicing at low intensity with emphasis on technique
- Practicing at high intensity
- Tapering
- Competing

The cycles that occur throughout the year are called *macrocycles*, and within each macrocycle the athlete will undergo microcycles that vary from week to week. It's also not surprising to see a substantial amount of overlap within each cycle. Many athletes like to include aerobic training and low intensity practice during their strengthening phase and vice versa.

As a competitive athlete, you'll want to maintain some degree of basic aerobic conditioning throughout the year. You can accomplish this by doing any aerobic activity for a minimum of thirty minutes, three to four times per week. Always start your aerobic workout with a five-minute warm-up period followed by a level of activity that maintains a heart rate of 70% to 80% of your maximum predicted heart rate (220 minus your age). You will want to leave enough time at the end of your work out for at least a five-minute cool down.

As you enter a more demanding phase of your training program, you can gradually increase the intensity and duration of your workouts by adding some endurance workouts and interval training. Keep in mind that as you increase the length of your workouts, your bones and joints will experience more stress. You can decrease the amount of physical stress to your body by doing low impact exercises like cycling or the elliptical trainer. This is particularly important for sports that require high levels of repetitive impact because too much impact can lead to stress fractures and other serious injuries. Examples of high impact sports include basketball, volleyball, tennis, and long-distance running.

Don't Just Lie There

Sooner or later you'll have an injury, and you won't want to let all your hard work go to waste. Let's use Joe, a seventeen-year-old basketball player, to demonstrate how to implement a well-rounded fitness program while recovering from an injury. Over the past few years Joe's been playing intense, year-round basketball in community leagues as well as at school. His goal was to play well at school, but he missed most of his sophomore season because of a stress fracture that he developed from doing too much high impact exercise. It didn't take long for Joe to realize that this unscheduled break was long overdue.

After several weeks of rest and recovery, Joe was starting to get some renewed enthusiasm about playing basketball. Although he wasn't ready to start running, his physician allowed him to ride the stationary bike. This allowed him to start some aerobic training without stressing his bones.

Joe figured that he had five months before preseason practice, and he would have to be ready to do at least one hour of high intensity activity by that time. He also knew that it would be eight weeks before he could start running and jumping on his broken leg.

When he started back to his workouts, he was amazed at how quickly he had gotten out of shape. He began a basic program of twenty minutes every other day with a goal of gradually increasing his workouts to include thirty minutes of moderate intensity aerobic exercise four times a week over the first month. Joe also started a light upper body-strengthening program including some calisthenics to strengthen his abs and torso.

During the second month, he gradually increased his workouts to forty-five minutes of light intensity aerobic activity twice a week with an additional thirty minutes of moderate to high intensity interval training twice a week. He also got permission to use the StairMaster during the second month so he could do some low impact weight-bearing exercise.

During the third month, he was able to start a walk-jog program on alternate days and continued increasing his nonweight-bearing, high intensity training so that by the end of the month, he was up to an hour twice a week.

By this point, Joe has regained most of his aerobic conditioning without stressing his overstressed bones. He has progressed from a nonweight-bearing program to a low impact program, and he is ready to start acclimating to the high impact demands of running and jumping on the basketball court. During the fourth month, he'll gradually introduce impact activities by running twice a week on soft surfaces like the beach or the track. In addition, he will try some jumping on soft sand or jumping up onto a foot-high landing so as not to stress his bones as he lands.

By the fifth month, Joe has increased his high impact conditioning program to three times a week and has begun to practice on a wood court. By the end of the month he'll be ready for the demands of preseason practice. Next year Joe is going to plan several periods of relative rest and recovery throughout the year. He's also going to be sure to vary his training program to include some low impact aerobic conditioning as a way to stay in shape without stressing his bones and joints.

CHAPTER 4

The Stronger Athlete

The stronger athlete will have a definite advantage in most sports. In this chapter, we'll see how a well-structured strengthening program can help you avoid injury and improve performance. We'll also discuss some of the limitations of strength training and review the best approaches to developing both sports specific strength and overall physical strength.

Establish a Strength Training Goal That Is Right for Your Sport

One of the first things that come to mind when you talk about strength training is a big, muscle-bound jock that rips his shirt apart every time they flex. Although strength training can increase the size of your muscles, the practical goal for most athletes is not to build bulky muscles but to increase strength, power, and endurance. Depending on your needs, you can design a resistance-training program that helps you achieve three basic results: hypertrophy (bigger muscles), maximal strength gains, and dynamic strength gains.

Your strength training goals will depend on the demands of your sport. Activities like power lifting, the shot put, and some positions in football require athletes to perform occasional maximal-strength maneuvers. Most sports, however, require the ability to generate power at a variety of workloads. A shot put, for example, requires an all-out, maximal effort with a sixteen-pound metal ball, whereas a baseball player may need to generate a substantial amount of power with a ball that only weighs a few ounces. This ability to generate power at a variety of workloads is referred to as *dynamic strength* and is the strength most athletes want to be focusing on.

In addition to dynamic strength, most sports require balanced strength development. Whether you're swinging a tennis racket or throwing a punch, you'll get the best results when your entire body is working in a coordinated effort to perform the task. To achieve this goal, you'll need to develop dynamic strength in your torso and upper body as well as your extremities. Overdevelopment of a particular muscle group with weak supportive and opposing muscle groups can lead to suboptimal performance and injury. For most athletes, the main strength-training goal is to develop balanced, dynamic strength throughout their body.

Now that you've defined your goal, we can talk about how you can get the best results. You can improve your strength and power by doing resistance training, plyometrics, and sprint training.

Resistance Training

The traditional approach to getting bigger and stronger utilizes free weights in a number of different patterns and sequences. Free weights are relatively inexpensive, they are adaptable to a variety of exercises, and they require a relatively small amount of storage space. Most experienced strength-training athletes and coaches use free weights as the core of their strengthening programs.

Using weight machines can complement your free-weight program by helping you isolate specific muscle groups. Some weight machines, like the lat pull-down machine, have the additional advantage of using pulleys to change the direction of resistance, allowing you to work in the opposite direction of gravity. Although some brands of resistance-training machines offer specific advantages, such as easy storage or a modified resistance method, you shouldn't expect to see a huge difference in your strength gains because you are using a fancy machine.

For the novice weight lifter, a properly designed weight machine can offer an added degree of safety by minimizing the risk of losing control of the weight and eliminating the need for a spotter's assistance when working out. Not withstanding the above, you can still hurt yourself if you take the wrong approach. You can decrease your chances of getting hurt by letting a certified trainer help you get acquainted with the equipment.

A good strength-training coach can help you set up a program that utilizes free weights and machines in a way that is appropriate for your needs. They can help you learn good technique and help you to decide when to push hard as well as when to back off.

There are several associations that certify strength and fitness trainers. The most respected include:

- The American College of Sports Medicine (ACSM)
- The National Strength and Conditioning Association (NSCA)
- The National Athletic Trainers' Association (NATA)

If you can't find a certified trainer, you'll want to be sure that your coach has some experience working with people that have similar training needs and that they know some of the concepts outlined in this chapter.

A good trainer can safely guide you through the various stages of your strength-training program. The first step of any program is to become familiar with the exercises by learning the proper timing and execution of the lifts. Most of the strength gains that you'll see during the first twelve weeks of your program are not because you are really getting stronger, but because of improved neuromuscular coordination—learning to coordinate the efficient recruitment of muscle fibers during the lift.

Since this type of coordination is the key benefit of the first part of your program, you can understand why there's no rush to start pushing heavy weights. You'll get the best results by using a resistance level that allows you to do your workout in a relatively safe and comfortable manner.

One way to select the amount of resistance is to select a weight that you can comfortably execute three to five sets of twelve to fifteen repetitions. If you can't make it to three sets of twelve then you need to decrease the weight. If you can comfortably finish five sets of fifteen, you're ready to advance to a slightly heavier weight. Using this high volume approach, with special attention to proper timing, breathing, and technique, will help you achieve your initial goal of learning good technique and developing neuromuscular coordination.

Coincidentally, the high volume approach also addresses the next goal of most strength-training programs: hypertrophy or bigger muscles. The most efficient way to increase muscle size is with low intensity workouts and volumes in the range of three to ten sets of eight to twelve repetitions. Your body adapts to the heavier forces by increasing the amount of muscle fiber as well as increasing muscle protein that makes up the fiber.

Your muscles aren't the only part of your body that responds to the challenge. When you do resistance training, you'll also strengthen your tendons, ligaments, and bones.

Once you've developed some neuromuscular coordination and hypertrophy, you're ready to advance your program. You can do this by using a slightly lower volume yet increasing the intensity of your workouts. A basic strength program would utilize loads that would allow you to complete three to five sets of four to six repetitions. This type of resistance program will begin to help you achieve significant maximal strength gains.

You can achieve maximal power gains by using high intensity, low-volume workouts with loads that would allow you to complete three to five sets of three reps. You need to be very cautious when using heavy loads. Insufficient preparation, improper technique, and poor supervision can lead to injury, and injuries are associated with the lowest rate of strength gains.

Another important safety issue is to always have an *experienced, attentive* spotter (or two) when you're going to lift heavy loads, particularly if the load can fall onto your body. Before you get your spotters in place, you'll want to warm up. A good approach is to warm up with a lighter weight yet using the same timing and technique that you will use while lifting the heavier weight.

You may want to take a brief reality break before you get carried away and start bench-pressing your neighbor's pickup truck. The strength-training goal for most athletes is not necessarily massive hypertrophy or maximal strength but rather the ability to generate power at a variety of workloads. As you already know, this is referred to as *dynamic strength*. This is the kind of strength that you need for sports like baseball, tennis, volleyball, basketball, Jiu-Jitsu, and soccer, to name a few.

Several researchers have shown that training with high repetitions and high intensity, along with workloads approximating 30%RM (repetition maximum— the maximal amount of weight that you can lift in a single try of that activity) produces the best dynamic strength development (Wilson 1993; Moss 1997). If your primary athletic focus is not powerlifting or bodybuilding, working with lighter workloads is safer and more adaptable to a demanding training program.

In each of these scenarios, I've referred to the level of intensity as a variable that can help you to achieve a specific result. Intensity can be defined as force multiplied by velocity. At a given weight, you can vary the intensity by adjusting the speed at which you lift the weight. In the initial stages of your strengthening program, your focus should be on developing good technique and coordination. The speed at which you lift a given weight should be relatively slow at first, and the timing of your lift phase should closely approximate the duration of the return phase. As you become more experienced, you can begin to shorten your lift phase by increasing the speed at which you lift the weight.

Breathe

Breathing is an important part of your lifting routine and should be coordinated with the timing of your lift. The best approach is to inhale as you bring the weight to the starting position, and then exhale during the last two thirds of your lift phase. You can inhale again as you return the weight to the initial position. Try to avoid holding your breath during the lift phase as this will unnecessarily increase your blood pressure and result in less than efficient oxygen exchange.

Hyperventilation (breathing rapidly) prior to lifting then holding your breath during the lift can decrease the blood supply to your brain and can lead to loss of consciousness. Needless to say, passing out while trying to lift a heavy weight is not a good idea. Hyperventilation prior to any exercise *does not* increase your blood oxygen level and should be avoided.

Training Systems

Plyometrics is a training system that utilizes an initial loading or stretching of a muscle group followed by a rapid contraction of the same muscle group. During the loading phase, the targeted muscle group must absorb the force being applied as it is lengthening (eccentric contraction, see definitions). Once the muscle group is loaded, it must quickly change direction and perform a concentric contraction. Repeated jumps are a good example of how your leg muscles absorb the downward force during the landing, then quickly change direction during the next jump.

Most plyometric exercises involving the lower extremities utilize some form of hopping or jumping with an exaggerated range of motion. You can perform plyometric exercises with your torso and upper extremities by using a medicine ball. Exercise with this heavy ball requires your upper body to absorb the momentum of the ball as you catch it before you redirect the muscle contraction to throw it back to your training partner.

In addition to adding variety to your workout program, plyometric exercises are an effective way of increasing strength and power. This form of exercise is typically more dynamic than weight training because you are challenging your muscles to work in a coordinated fashion. Plyometric drills can also help you to develop skills that you can carry over to your primary sport because they require good balance and coordination. When properly performed, plyometric exercises may improve body mechanics, decrease landing forces, and hopefully decrease injures (Hewett 1996).

There are a few things to keep in mind to avoid hurting yourself while performing plyometrics. Typically these drills should not be introduced until after you've completed several months of basic conditioning, and they should only be performed after a good ten to fifteen minutes of warm-up. Be sure to get an experienced trainer to help you with technique, and as with most other training tools, be sure to start easy and build up slowly.

Sprints

Many sports require an occasional all-out effort for relatively short distances, and one of the best ways to improve your speed is to perform sprint training. Most sprinting drills involve running, but you can also perform sprints that challenge other muscle groups by using a bicycle, rowing machine, or swimming pool.

Your goal is to perform short, high intensity sprints with a full recovery between each interval. You can monitor your heart rate to make sure that you are at least below 100 beats per minute before you get started on the next sprint. A good recovery will ensure that you are ready to challenge your anaerobic power system by giving it your all on the next sprint. On the other hand, if you take shorter recovery period with lower intensity sprints, you will get more of an aerobic/anaerobic challenge.

As with plyometric training, you'll want to wait until you've done a couple of months of basic conditioning before you start any serious sprint training. You'll also want to be sure to include plenty of time for a good warm-up and cooldown every time you perform a sprint workout.

With the help of your trainer, you can design a strength-training program that fits your training cycles. There is no specific strength-training program that is right for every athlete, and an individual athlete may need to alter his or her strength-training program as they move from one phase of their training cycle to another. Depending on your needs, you can design a program to maintain and improve your strength while you are off-season or taking a break from your primary sport.

You might take a couple of months during your off-season to work on hypertrophy. As you get closer to preseason practice, you can gradually transition to a program that focuses on maximal strength gains. When preseason practice begins, you may continue your strengthening program but focus on developing dynamic strength.

The volume and intensity of your strengthening workouts should complement the amount of training you do in your primary sport. As you start to train harder in your primary sport, you can back off on the volume and intensity of your strength training. When you get closer to competition, you'll want stick to light workouts and spend most of your time and energy focusing on the specifics of your primary sport.

Strengthen Specific Body Parts

If your sport stresses specific body parts, you can take advantage of the off-season to strengthen those body parts and supporting structures. A tennis player might want to focus on a shoulder-strengthening program whereas a cyclist might use weights to strengthen her legs. Depending on the demands of your sport, you can focus on maximal strength or dynamic strength. A cyclist who specializes in sprints might focus on maximal strength as opposed to a long-distance cyclist who might focus on dynamic strength.

Develop Dynamic Strength Throughout Your Body

During most of your training cycles, you'll want to devote some time and energy to maintaining dynamic strength throughout your body. You already know that the best way to do this is by using lighter workloads but with a more intense lift and constant acceleration of the weight. Because of the important role that your torso plays in stabilizing your upper body, you'll want to be sure to include some torso-strengthening exercises on a regular basis.

There are a variety of ways to design a full body-strengthening program, and your approach will depend on your needs as well as your overall training load. A common approach focuses on one aspect of your body one day and another part the next day. With this type of approach, you can fully stress a particular area of your body and allow it to recover the next day while you are challenging a different part of your body. A sample program might look like this:

M	T	W	Th	F	S	S
Chest & Back	Legs	Arms & Torso	Rest	Chest & Back	Legs & Torso	Rest

The intensity of your workouts can vary from day to day. To allow for adequate recovery, you can follow a heavy workout with a light day or a rest day. You may want to consider doing only one heavy workout with a given body part each week. You can follow up later in the week with a lighter workout of the same area. Alternately, you could do two heavy chest and back workouts with lighter leg and torso workout one week. The following week you can do light chest and back workouts with a couple of heavy leg and torso workouts. Again, the key is to combine moderate stress with adequate recovery.

A second approach to full body strengthening is to use supersets. This approach involves completing a series of sets using exercises that stress different body parts. A workout might begin with crunches followed by lat pull-downs, biceps curls, triceps extension, leg extensions, bench press, rowing, and leg curls. Once you've finished the first set, you might want to stretch for a short break if you are using heavier weights or move right into the next set if you are working with lighter weights. This approach will allow you to work out your entire body in a short amount of time. You can do two to three light supersets per week when your time and energy are focused on your primary sport.

Correcting Imbalances

Muscles work in opposing pairs to move and stabilize your body during activity. Opposing muscle groups typically work in the opposite direction, such as biceps and triceps on your arms or the hamstrings and quadriceps in your thighs. Certain sports favor the development of one side of the pair more than the other, and the resulting imbalance can lead to poor body mechanics and injury. Let's take the example of a long-distance runner to illustrate this point. Running primarily utilizes the lower body and develops relatively stronger, tighter hamstrings and lower back muscles with relatively weaker quadriceps and abdominal muscles. An athlete whose primary sport is running will want to consider a light strength-training program to strengthen his quads and abs.

Recovering from an Injury

Hopefully, it won't take an injury to get you to identify and correct the uneven muscle development associated with your sport. A qualified physical therapist or athletic trainer can help you develop a strength-training program that addresses your specific situation.

Once you suffer from an injury, you don't have to lie around and get flabby while you recover. You'll get so out of shape that you will reinjure yourself when you get back into your sport. Depending on the nature of the injury, you can make good use of your recovery time by using a strength-training program to stay in shape. This will make your transition back to a demanding training program much easier and will prevent further injury as you increase the training load.

Strength Training for Women Too

Just in case you were wondering, everything we've talked about applies to women as well as men. Women respond to resistance training with similar percentages of strength gains and hypertrophy as men. In general, the process and principles of strength training appear to be independent of gender (Barrett 1990).

Strength training is an attractive choice for all women. Although it's rapidly becoming the exception, there are still situations where young girls don't get the same amount of physical challenge as boys do. With a limited training background, some girls won't have the same relative amount of strength and coordination as boys do. As more women enter recreational and competitive sports programs, the benefits of developing full body-dynamic strength may be even more important for women than their male counterparts.

In addition to increasing muscle mass and strength, resistance training also improves bone density. *Osteoporosis* is the common thinning and weakening of the bones that occurs in women as they age. It can lead to deformities, pain, and disability. Your bone mass will peak in early adulthood, and your peak bone density is an important predictor of future bone strength.

Because of all of its potential health benefits, strength training is a highly recommended addition to any woman's fitness program.

Strength Training in Children

Despite all the controversy as to the safety and efficacy of strength training in children, some parents still want to get a jump on the competition by starting their child's strength-training program early in life. *Before the onset of puberty, most of the apparent strength gains are related to improved coordination and not to actual strength gains.* That is to say, the child learns how to lift the weight in a coordinated and efficient manner.

Although strength training in the preadolescent period doesn't make kids stronger, it's reasonable to expect that a child that is familiar with the techniques of strength training may have some advantage after they hit puberty. It can be argued that familiarity might offer an advantage to a child that wants to be involved in competitive weight lifting and that familiarity is less important in sports that require dynamic strength.

Safety is the biggest concern for kids who want to lift weights. Injuries frequently result from carelessness and trying to lift more weight than the child can handle. Good training and supervision are essential. Since most of the benefit from strength training is from improved coordination, the primary focus should be on learning the proper technique and not on lifting heavy weights.

As the child starts to lift heavier weights, the chance of losing control of the weight increases. Even if the weight doesn't fall on them, the pressures of an unbalanced load can easily injure a young athlete. Placing heavy loads on young bones can cause growth plate injuries as well as lower back injuries. Both can have serious long-term effects on the child's health.

David Webb (Webb 1990) has outlined eleven important points to consider when young athletes are involved in strength training. They are summarized below:

1. The child should consider weight training to be worthwhile, and only continue if it is fun, satisfying, and safe.
2. The child should be mature enough to be coachable, and a certified strength training coach that is familiar with working with children should be consulted. Close supervision is essential with a student to instructor ratio of less than ten to one.
3. The child should have medical clearance to do weight training.

4. All parties involved should pay close attention to any joint or back pain and consult a physician for any severe pains or pains that do not resolve in two days.

5. Because of the developmental lag in shoulder, abdominal wall, and trunk muscles and the high incidence of shoulder and back overuse injuries, the child should begin with a *prehabilitation* program that strengthens these areas. Prehabilitation is a preventive exercise program that strengthens muscles that are vulnerable to injury before they are injured. Rehabilitation occurs after muscles are injured.

6. Submaximal exercises that focus on strength and endurance should be utilized instead of pure strength exercises. Exercises should be done in three to four sets of ten to twenty reps. If the child cannot perform a minimum of three sets of ten reps, then the weight is probably too heavy, whereas, if the child can complete twenty reps, then they are ready for the next weight increase. On each set, fatigue, not failure, is the desired goal.

7. Resistance exercises should be done through a full range of motion.

8. Strict attention should be paid to maintaining a normal curvature of the lower spine during any exercise in which compression loads are placed on the spine. Exercises such as straight-leg dead lifts and good mornings (lifting a barbell while bending forward at the hips) that involve both compression loading and flexion or torsion of the lower back should be avoided.

9. Training should be limited to three days per week.

10. Exercises for all muscle groups should be included, and there should be a good balance between exercises for opposing muscle groups.

11. Training should be advanced in small increments with respect to both the amount of resistance used and the motor skills required.

Even though the onset of puberty will bring on substantial strength gains from weight training, the importance of safety and supervision continue to be essential. It's common for young athletes to compete in the weight room to see who can lift the most with a single repetition. They also tend to focus on the "mirror muscles" such as their biceps, pects, abs, and quads. The focus needs to be redirected to balanced muscle development and core strengthening (Loud 2003). Again, the high volume, low resistance approach is the best way to develop hypertrophy and dynamic strength.

Be Careful

Hopefully the information in this chapter will serve as a good introduction to strength training. I encourage you to find a certified strength-training coach to help you develop a program based on your age, sport, and level of competition. A good coach will teach you safe, conservative approaches to getting stronger and hopefully keep you off the injured list.

CHAPTER 5

Challenging Environments

Whether you are a top-notch athlete who competes for a living or a part-time, recreational athlete, sooner or later, you're going to need to compete in harsh environmental conditions. Some athletes may have to deal with multiple extremes in one day. Triathletes, for example, could risk hypothermia during the cold water swim, then suffer from heat exhaustion a couple of hours later during the run. If the event were held at high altitude, you might have to endure acute mountain sickness as well.

In this chapter, we'll see how environmental conditions can affect your performance and how you can do your best to be prepared for the worst conditions.

Variations in Temperature

Your body is so well tuned that your performance will begin to suffer if your core temperature deviates more than a few degrees in either direction. Larger deviations in core temperature will affect your judgment and jeopardize your safety. To complicate matters, you might be on an exposed mountainside with subzero temperatures or on a running trail five miles from the nearest road on a 95-degree day.

Since both hypothermia and heat exhaustion can affect your judgment, you'll need to be able to recognize dangerous conditions while you can still make the right decisions. The best approach is to take the proper preventive measures and be keenly aware of the signs that you may be having difficulty adapting.

Heat

Working muscles can increase your baseline heat production by a factor of twenty, so staying cool while exercising in warm weather becomes a challenge.

To keep your body within its optimal temperature range, you'll need to move warm blood from your hardworking muscles to where it can cool off at your skin. Once the warm blood makes it to your skin, you can begin to dissipate heat through three physical mechanisms: radiation, conduction, and evaporation. Your ability to dissipate heat by these factors depends on your level of physiologic adaptation, the environmental conditions, and your clothing. Let's take a look at how you can maximize the cooling effect of each of these factors.

Physiological Adaptation

With gradual training in warm weather, your body will initiate the adaptations that make exercise in the heat possible. Most of the changes are centered on the management of fluids, and athletes that are acclimated to the heat will automatically store more fluid in between each workout. Having more fluid will improve their ability to circulate blood to their peripheral tissues and allow the athlete to perspire at the first sign of heat stress.

The process of acclimatization begins within a few days of training in a warmer environment and most of the adaptations are complete after one week. Even if it is cool out, you can start to prepare for warm conditions by doing some endurance training. Longer workouts, even in cooler conditions, will help you start making some of the physiological adaptations that you'll need for warmer conditions.

The length of time that it takes to adapt to a hot environment varies. It may take up to two weeks of training in warm conditions to achieve near-maximal acclimatization (Terrados 1995, Binkley 2002). Further changes that decrease sodium losses in sweat may take up to six weeks (Guyton 1996). It may take you even longer to adapt if you've spent most of your life in a cool climate.

Although it can take weeks and even months to acclimate to exercise in warm environments, your level of heat acclimatization will begin to diminish after only six days in a cool environment (Binkley 2002). A well-prepared athlete needs to anticipate challenging conditions when an upcoming event will occur in a warm climate, season, or time of day. Some events, like the Hawaiian Ironman, are purposely held in challenging environmental conditions so it should be no surprise that the heat will be a factor.

Being prepared for a surprise heat wave can be more of a problem. That's why so many heat injuries occur during the spring when athletes haven't had an opportunity to acclimate to hot weather. I had some firsthand experience managing some heatstroke patients while attending a 10-kilometer race on Catalina Island in March. One of the competitors became disoriented after running up a long hill only three miles into the race, and by the time the paramedics got him to the emergency room, he had a core temperature of 106°F. Fortunately, he received immediate medical attention and was released from the hospital the next day with no major complications, although after several years of follow up, he still has difficulty handling hot conditions. Most people who have had heat exhaustion or heatstroke need to be aware that they are at higher risk of heat injury with subsequent heat challenges.

You can improve your ability to tolerate the heat by properly scheduling your training program. Having to compete in the middle of a hot day can be a problem if you usually train in the morning while it's cool. As part of your strategy, you can move some of your training sessions to the middle of the day when it is warmer, or you can wear heavier clothing while training in cool weather. As you start to train in warmer conditions, you'll need to lower the intensity and duration of your workouts to give your body a chance to adapt.

If you are thinking that doing all of your workouts in the heat is a good idea, you need to keep in mind that it probably won't improve your performance in cool weather. Furthermore, the added physiological burden of training in the heat will limit the amount of time you can spend performing drills that will improve your technique. It will also take you longer to recover from an exhausting workout in the heat when compared to a similar workout in a comfortable environment. Having said that, you still need to consider doing some workouts in the heat if you anticipate that you'll be called to action when the weather is hot.

Many of the adaptive factors that improve your performance in hot conditions require optimal hydration. Remember that good hydration is what allows you to move heat from the core of your body to your skin and without perspiration you'll lose the cooling effects of evaporation. You'll be maximizing your ability to perform in the heat if you make a conscious effort to stay hydrated before, during, and after your strenuous workouts.

It is important to anticipate dehydration because your thirst mechanism won't remind you to drink until you've lost enough fluid to adversely affect your performance. Even if water is available, most athletes will only replace half of their fluid losses unless they are prompted to drink by some source other than thirst. This means that if you wait until you are thirsty to start drinking, you'll have to assimilate over a quart of fluid to get back to your baseline. Needless to say, trying to down a quart of fluid in the heat of competition is a poor solution because your ability to absorb fluids is compromised when you are dehydrated and overheated. To further complicate matters, over-hydrating can also get you into serious problems with bloating and electrolyte disturbances.

Since it is so important, I am going to go over it one more time. The smarter athlete will have a predetermined fluid strategy and they will set a goal of drinking a measured amount of fluid in a given time period. Ideally, your fluid intake should balance but not exceed your sweat losses. You can estimate your fluid losses by weighing yourself before and after performing a workout. If you keep track of how much fluid you drank during the workout, you'll be able to calculate how much more you need to drink to stay fully hydrated during a similar workout in the future.

Let's take the example of a seventeen-year-old basketball player that weighs 150 pounds before a typical game and 146 pounds after the game. If she drank a quart of fluid (a quart of water weighs approximately two pounds), we can calculate that she lost a total of six pounds of fluid and replaced only two. The four-pound fluid deficit means that she is over 2% dehydrated (4/150=0.027). At this level of dehydration, her performance will start to decline. To be at her best throughout the entire game, she'll need to increase her total fluid intake for the game to two to three quarts. Since this is a lot of fluid, she'll need to spread her intake throughout the game to keep from getting bloated. You can make similar estimates of your fluid losses for a variety of conditions so you know how much to drink while practicing and competing under similar circumstances.

By staying optimally hydrated during practice, you'll not only get the most out of your practice sessions, you'll also get a jump on your recovery for the next day's practice. If you're dehydrated and overheated, you'll have trouble recovering from your tough workouts, and you'll be showing up at the next day's workout feeling flat and lethargic.

Fluid Deprivation

The all-too-common practice of fluid deprivation during practice and training has no basis in science.

The adaptations that allow you to function in the heat become ineffective if you are dehydrated, and it's fairly clear that there is no adaptation to dehydration (Terrados 1995). To the contrary, athletes should be conditioning themselves to drink at appropriate levels so they can get used to training and competing while drinking optimal amounts of fluid.

Now that you know how much to drink we can talk about what type of fluid works best. Water works well when you exercise for less than one to two hours, but a sports drink with a small amount of carbohydrate (approximately 6% to 8%) may improve your performance even during short periods of exercise. Using a sports drink may also help you to increase your fluid intake because drinking plain water may decrease your thirst level before you've completely rehydrated (Maughan 1993).

If you are going to be exercising for longer than two hours, you'll want to replace your fluid losses with a sports drink containing carbohydrates and electrolytes. Even though conditioned athletes lose only small amounts of sodium in their sweat, these losses can add up over time and using water alone can get you into trouble (Wexler 2002). You can keep from getting low on sodium and potassium by choosing from a variety of sports drinks. You will want to try the different types of sports drinks during practice to see which one you like the most.

Avoid salt tablets, fluids containing alcohol or caffeine, and medications that affect urine output or perspiration. These include many over-the-counter cold and flu remedies. If you are sick, you should avoid heavy exertion, and you should not train at all if you are running a fever. Since illness and medication can have multiple effects on your body, you should always consult your family doctor to see if it is safe to exercise with your condition.

Regardless of how well acclimated you are, you'll still need to maintain a great deal of respect for hot conditions. This means adjusting the intensity and duration of your workouts and under most circumstances, not trying to set a record when conditions are particularly hot and/or humid. Your competition will be facing the same conditions, and they will be making similar adjustments. Furthermore, we will see that regardless of how well hydrated and conditioned you are, there are conditions when it is too hot or humid to exercise. Heat injuries can have long-term effects on your future performance, and it seems that every year some well-conditioned athlete dies from heatstroke.

Physical Factors

Once you've moved the heat to the surface of your body and created enough sweat to wet your skin, you're ready to start cooling off. You can take advantage of four basic cooling mechanisms: conduction, convection, evaporation, and radiation. Convection and evaporation are the most effective ways to lose heat (Lugo-Amador 2004). To cool down you'll need to conduct heat from your warm body to the air around you. As long as the air temperature around you is lower than your body temperature, you can transfer heat from your body to the environment. Eventually, as the layer of air around you warms up, the rate of conduction will slow down.

This is the point where you need convection to move the warm air away from your skin and replace it with cooler air. This is what happens as you move around or as the wind blows past your body. The greater the wind speed, the better the cooling effect. To maximize conduction and convection, you'll want to avoid clothing that traps warm air around your body. Clothes that are slightly wet will increase cooling because wet clothing increases the amount of conductive heat loss by a rate of five times that of dry clothing (Bracker 1992).

Once the environmental temperature equals your body temperature, conduction stops and environmental temperatures above your body temperature will actually make you warmer. Even at temperatures equal to or above your body temperature, you can still get substantial cooling from evaporation, but the effectiveness of evaporation as a cooling mechanism is directly related to the level of humidity. As the humidity becomes more than 60%, your ability to lose heat through evaporation deteriorates and as the ambient humidity approaches 100%, the rate of evaporation approaches zero. That's why exercise in hot, humid conditions is more of a physiologic challenge than exercising at a similar temperature with lower humidity. I've included a heat index in Table 5.1 so that you can get an idea of how humidity affects your overall heat exposure.

		HEAT INDEX							
T				**Percent Humidity**					
E	**20**	**30**	**40**	**50**	**60**	**70**	**80**	**90**	**100**
M	115	120	135	151					
P	110	112	123	137	150				
E	105	105	113	123	135	149			
R	100	99	104	110	120	132	144		
A	95	93	96	101	107	114	124	136	
T	90	87	90	93	96	100	106	113	122
U	85	82	84	86	88	90	93	97	102	108
R	80	77	78	79	81	82	85	86	88	91
E	75	72	73	74	75	76	77	78	79	80
°F	70	66	67	68	69	70	70	71	71	72

80°F–90°F Fatigue with prolonged exposure and/or physical activity.

90°F–105°F Heatstroke/heat exhaustion possible with prolonged exposure or physical activity.

105°F–130°F Heatstroke or heat exhaustion likely with prolonged exposure or physical activity.

>130°F Heatstroke likely with continued exposure.

The Heat Index is a specialized way of assessing the combined effect of temperature and humidity. These calculations are assuming shade and light wind. You'll need to add 15° if you are going to be exposed to direct sunlight.

Table 5.1 Heat Index.

In addition to conduction and evaporation, your body can exchange heat with the environment through radiation. Your body radiates heat in all directions and absorbs radiant heat from the sun and the objects that surround you. Cloud cover, shade, hats, and clothing can all decrease the warming effects of radiant heat from the sun. The other major source of radiant heat is your training surface. Hot asphalt, concrete, or sand can radiate a substantial amount of heat so on hot days, you may want to train on grass or shaded training surfaces.

Some athletes try to stay cool by spraying themselves with cold water or soaking themselves with a cold, wet sponge. Although this may feel refreshing, it probably does little to effectively lower your core temperature (ACSM, Armstrong 1996). Placing any extremely cold substance on your skin can cause your capillaries to constrict and may actually undermine your body's cooling mechanisms.

In the same manner, drinking cold fluids may feel good, and they may absorb some heat from your body, but cold fluids will also slow your rate of fluid absorption. If you want for optimal cooling and absorption, it is recommended that you drink fluid that is between 60°F and 70°F (ACSM, Costill 1996).

Since you are trying to get rid of heat, it makes sense to avoid adding any heat. Getting into the shade as frequently as possible as well as wearing light-colored clothing can help you avoid the effects of radiant heat. Wearing a hat can protect you from radiant heat, and you'll get plenty of conductive and evaporative heat loss if it's designed so that air can get through it.

Although helmets can retain heat, a well-designed helmet can cool you with air circulation plus block radiant heat from the sun. Additionally, properly designed helmets are more aerodynamic. In sports like cycling, you'll do less work to travel at the same speed. The result is that in some circumstances, wearing a helmet is actually cooler than not wearing one.

Your brain is your best protection from heat-related illness. Table 5.2 presents how to identify and treat overheating.

You can protect yourself from waking up in the hospital, wondering what happened by:

• Being acclimated before training and competing in the heat
• Properly hydrating before, during, and after exercise
• Staying cool during the last twelve hours before competition
• Wearing the right clothing and equipment
• Recognizing potentially dangerous conditions and adjusting your level of exertion
• Recognizing that no matter how well-conditioned and hydrated you are, there are still some conditions that make exercise and competition a bad idea

The effects of overheating can manifest themselves in a variety of ways:

cramps*	headache	difficulty with coordination
dizziness*	nausea	
fainting*	vomiting	chills and goose bumps
fatigue		

*Early stages

Treatment

By identifying and treating the problem in the early stages, you can prevent serious complications.

1. Stop the activity and get the athlete to a cool surface in the shade if possible.
2. While you are waiting for help to arrive, drinking cool liquid (60°F–70°F) can help as long as the athlete is alert and talking.
3. You can increase the amount of evaporative heat loss by keeping the athlete wet and by fanning them. Lightweight, wet clothing has five times the cooling effect of dry skin, allowing you to keep the athletes clothes on as long as they don't have insulating layers.
4. Any insulating clothes such as jackets, windbreakers, sweats, hats, or helmets should be removed.
5. Cold, wet towels with ice packs can be placed in the back of the neck and under the armpits.
6. Immersion in cool water is an effective cooling mechanism as long as the athlete is not at risk for drowning from loss of consciousness or cramps.

Table 5.2 How to identify and treat overheating.

The Other Extreme: Prolonged Cold

Hypothermia, frostbite, and death are all potential complications of prolonged cold exposure. In addition to jeopardizing your health, hypothermia will adversely affect your motor skills, strength, aerobic performance, and cognitive performance (Murray 1995). Your best protection from becoming a human icicle is to be aware of potentially dangerous conditions and be prepared with the right kind of equipment and support. Let's explore some of the factors that affect your ability to perform well in cold environments.

Surprise!

Most people don't get up in the morning planning to get hypothermia. Frequently, it's an unexpected event that results in prolonged exposure to dangerously cold conditions. A change in weather, car problems, or getting lost or injured in the wilderness can be disastrous if you're not prepared. It doesn't have to be extremely cold for you to get hypothermic. Even seemingly mild conditions like running a marathon on a breezy 76°F day can result in hypothermia. This is because your body performs best at approximately 98°F to 100°F. If you are surrounded by air that is twenty degrees cooler than this optimal range, heat lost from your body will exceed the heat it generates by exercise.

An old proverb suggests that a smart person learns from their mistakes, but a wise person learns from someone else's mistakes. Learn from someone else's mistakes. Be aware of the potential for exposure and be prepared for the unexpected. Hypothermia is possible even during a swim meet in a heated, indoor pool. Ask yourself: What if? If you think that it won't happen to you, then you're definitely in the high-risk group.

Some of basic precautions to take before you venture from civilization include letting someone know where you are going and when you will be checking in to let him or her know that you are back. You should also check the weather forecast, but keep in mind that forecasters are frequently incorrect. You'll want to anticipate the potential for harsh conditions by carrying gear to keep you warm and dry in case something goes wrong. (See Table 5.3 for cold weather equipment.)

If you plan to venture into the cold, you're going to want the right clothing and equipment.

- The inner layers of your clothing should be designed to provide insulation yet be able to wick water away from your skin. Products made from polypropylene do not retain water to the same degree as wool or cotton and are a good choice for your inner layers.
- The middle layers should provide insulation without trapping water.
- The outer layer needs to protect you from wind and water but must still be able to breathe so that moisture doesn't get trapped inside your clothing.

New synthetic materials have maximized these properties, but be prepared to pay some serious prices for the best stuff. By carrying a waterproof pack you can add or remove layers as conditions change. This is a good way of keeping your inner layers dry when you perspire during periods of heavy exertion.

Table 5.3 Gear suited for cold-weather exercise.

It's a good idea to have extra food and water rations because nutrition and hydration are significant factors in your performance during prolonged cold exposure. During an emergency, your performance needs to be at its best because your life may depend on it.

Although you might be surrounded by cold, you can still have significant fluid losses from perspiration during intense exercise. You may not even notice that you are perspiring because in windy, dry conditions your sweat can evaporate so quickly that you won't notice it accumulating on your skin. Heavy breathing can also cause substantial fluid losses during cold, dry conditions. The mist that comes out of your mouth when you exhale on a cold day actually contains water from your respiratory tract, and during heavy exertion this water loss will add up.

Since dehydration in the cold will have a negative impact on your physical and mental performance, it's a good idea to bring along plenty of fluid if you are going to exercise in the cold. Try to keep your water or sports drink inside your protective gear so that it stays warm because cold fluids are absorbed slowly and will lower your body temperature.

Alcohol may give you a warming sensation because it dilates the vessels that go to your skin. Unfortunately, this will accelerate heat loss, and the diuretic effects of alcohol will also contribute to fluid losses. To make matters worse, alcohol will impair your judgment, and in an emergency you'll need to have all your brain cells working together.

As a final resort, you can also use clean snow or rainwater as a source of fluid in emergency situations. If you have to use snow, try to ingest it while you are on the move and generating heat instead of while you are resting.

Good nutrition is important under any circumstances. When it is cold, your body needs to burn more calories just to keep warm. When your blood sugar gets low, your physical and cognitive performance will decrease along with your ability to generate heat (Passias 1996). This can be a major problem if you're trying to stay warm.

Sports bars are a good source of highly concentrated calories, and they come in lightweight, airtight packages. You would be well-advised to stash a few of your favorite bars in your emergency kit and cold weather gear. While you are at it, throw in a few bars for your training partners.

The effects of cold weather become compounded when you're wet. This is true whether it is from perspiration, rain, or immersion. As with warm environments, evaporation of water from your skin will have a substantial cooling effect. Water is a better conductor of heat than air, and immersion in water will increase conductive heat losses by a factor of 25 (Bracker 1992). To complicate matters, the protective properties of your cold weather gear may diminish if they become wet. Having a plan for staying dry is an important part of being prepared for venturing into cold conditions. You may want to stash some lightweight, water-resistant gear in an airtight bag just in case you get soaked.

Wind will increase the cooling effect of cold weather because as it whips across your skin, it moves warm air away from your body and increases the rate of evaporation. Both of these factors can have a powerful effect on the total amount of heat that you lose. In the colder parts of the world, the ambient temperature is reported in absolute numbers as well as calculated for the wind chill factor. At -30°F, exposed skin will freeze in seconds, but with a 20 mph wind you can get rapid freezing at +10° F. With prolonged exposure your skin will freeze at temperatures as high as +28° F (-2° C) (Fritz 1989).

Once your skin is frozen, it's better to wait until you can get warm and stay warm before trying to rewarm your skin. Repeated freezing and warming is more harmful to your skin than prolonged freezing, because it is during the thawing process that damage to your skin occurs. It's better just to be prepared to cover all parts of your body, including your face, if you think that there is a chance of being exposed to this kind of weather.

Getting warmed up before exercise takes a little longer in cold weather because your circulatory system will keep warm blood toward the center of your body and away from your muscles. When you are resting, your muscles will help insulate you from the cold, but as you start to exercise, your body will begin to shunt blood to your muscles. This is fine as long as you keep moving and generating heat.

Once you stop exercising, you'll start to lose large amounts of heat, and your core temperature will fall rapidly. That's why intermittent exercise during cold conditions will cause hypothermia more rapidly than continuous exercise. If it's cold out, you're better off maintaining a sustainable pace than a pace that requires frequent rest periods.

You're probably wondering how to carry around so much of the stuff you need to protect yourself from the cold. One of the best solutions is to have a lightweight pack with a water bladder for your fluids and some extra compartments for basic survival supplies (Morton 2004). These include:

1. Fire making supplies: matches, lighter, and a small photo film container of petroleum jelly soaked cotton balls for tinder
2. A compass and topographical map of the area
3. Two large, industrial orange plastic bags for waterproofing, windproofing, and signaling
4. A solid knife with a grip and finger guard
5. A signaling mirror (with hole for aiming)
6. A whistle
7. Water purification tablets
8. A small, bright LED light for night vision and signaling
9. Sunglasses and sunscreen
10. Extra clothing, hat, and gloves
11. Food, carbohydrate bars
12. Surveyors tape for marking your path or signaling
13. First aid supplies

In summary, exercising in the cold can have a substantial effect on your performance and safety. Even though you can make some physiologic adaptations to the cold, you'll need to be prepared with the right equipment as well as plenty of food and water. If you frequently venture into the wilderness, you may want to look at some of the referenced articles or take a wilderness survival course. There are some things you can do to prepare against hypothermia. Table 5.4 shows some of the early signs of hypothermia and its treatment.

If you or one of your friends is beginning to show signs of hypothermia, you'll notice the following symptoms:

- Weakness
- Shivering
- Lethargy
- Slurred speech
- Dizziness
- Confusion
- Diarrhea
- Thirst

Warm fluids and carbohydrate replacements are a good idea if the person is conscious and talking. Dry clothing can increase insulation and help prevent further heat loss.

If you are stuck in a remote area away from emergency services, you need to STOP (Sit down, Think, Observe, and Plan). You will need to decide whether to shelter in place until help comes or whether to keep moving. If you have to move, it's better to keep moving toward help at a slow sustainable pace. If you can no longer continue to move and have to lie down, be sure to provide insulation from the cold ground using leaves or pine needles. If conditions are windy, try to get out of the wind. If it is snowing, you can consider making a snow cave as they can offer a substantial amount of protection from the elements. Upon arrival to civilization and while you wait for assistance, you can begin active rewarming with warm fluids or an electric blanket if one is available.

Table 5.4 First aid for hypothermia.

High Altitudes

Athletes of all ages and abilities are traveling to high altitudes to ski, backpack, or ride mountain bikes. Many athletes venture even higher to find untracked powder or ascend challenging peaks. Under all of these circumstances, high altitude can significantly affect your performance and safety.

To get a better understanding of what happens as you go to higher altitudes, it is helpful to understand what happens at sea level. At sea level the barometric pressure is 760 mm Hg (mercury) and the air is composed of approximately 21% oxygen, 78% nitrogen, and less than 1% carbon dioxide and water. Deep in your tissues, there is a relative lack of oxygen and excess of carbon dioxide. Simply put, the mission is to get the oxygen from the air to your tissues and the carbon dioxide from your tissues into the air.

Moving carbon dioxide out is a comparatively easy task because at the existing concentrations it is easily dissolved in the blood and released into the air. The more difficult task is to get the oxygen to the tissues. To achieve this goal, God created an incredible molecule called hemoglobin. Each hemoglobin molecule is capable of binding four oxygen molecules and delivering them to your tissues. At sea level, your hemoglobin has an optimal attraction for oxygen, and it captures the right amount in your lungs and releases the optimal amount in your tissues. So far, so good.

As you begin to climb, the barometric pressure begins to decrease, and you'll start to notice that there is less oxygen as you approach the 5,000-foot elevation. At this level, you have to breathe harder to get the same amount of oxygen and exercise performance begins to decrease. Fortunately, your hemoglobin can adapt to high altitudes and changes its affinity for oxygen, but this takes some time.

Most healthy individuals are able to safely tolerate exercise in range of 5,000 to 7,000 feet without acclimatization although performance may be decreased in sports that require high aerobic demands. *Caution is recommended for flatlanders who want to make all-out efforts at altitudes greater than 5,000 feet prior to acclimatization. This is particularly important for individuals with sickle cell trait. See Table 5.5.*

> Unlike sickle cell disease, a severely disabling condition in which the individual has inherited both genes for sickle cell disease, the person with sickle cell trait has only one gene for sickle cell disease and is not clinically affected by this condition. However, people with sickle cell trait are at increased risk of severe muscle damage, kidney failure, and even death if they rapidly ascend to altitude levels above 5,000 feet and perform high intensity exercise.
>
> A typical scenario would be that of an African American basketball player who travels from sea level to a college basketball tryout in Colorado. Being early in the season, he is a little out of shape yet he has got to go all-out to get on the team. Halfway through the tryout he collapses and has to be taken to the emergency room where they determine that he is in deep trouble due to severe muscle breakdown and imminent kidney failure.

Table 5.5 Sickle cell trait.

Severe muscle breakdown and kidney damage can occur in *any* individual at *any* altitude if they exercise at levels substantially beyond their ability. Being unaccustomed to the expected workload, rapidly ascending to high altitude and having sickle cell trait are all risk factors for this type of injury.

Before we start talking about how high altitude affects performance, let's look at what happens when you have difficulty adapting to a change in altitude. You won't be an expert in high altitude physiology after reading these paragraphs, so you'll have to do more preparation if you plan to travel above 12,000 feet. Unfortunately, since some people will run into serious trouble with altitudes above 8,000 feet, you'll want to have an idea about what can happen so that you can respond appropriately.

Approximately 15% to 30% of skiers who travel to Colorado ski resorts experience symptoms of *acute mountain sickness*. They include headache, fatigue, upset stomach, light-headedness, and difficulty sleeping. These would be bad symptoms to have if you were going to the mountains to play chess let alone engage in challenging physical activity. Clearly, if you were experiencing these symptoms it would be wise for you to stop your ascent and allow yourself to acclimate. As an alternative, you can descend 1,500 feet or until your symptoms have resolved. If you have had difficulty adapting in the past, you may want to consider talking to your doctor about a prescription medication that can help you adjust to high altitude.

Travelers that rapidly ascend to altitudes above 8,000 feet will increase their chances of developing *high altitude pulmonary edema* (HAPE). The higher and faster you climb, the greater the risk. The symptoms usually begin one to three nights after you have begun to ascend and are more common in those that are under twenty years old but can occur at any age. They include at least two of the following: shortness of breath at rest, cough, weakness, decreased exercise performance, chest tightness, or congestion.

High altitude cerebral edema (HACE) can occur in accelerated cases of acute mountain sickness and HAPE. One of the early signs of HACE is difficulty maintaining normal gait or inability to walk in a straight line. The symptoms can also include headache, severe weakness, confusion, altered consciousness, and coma. Like HAPE, the symptoms may present themselves one to three days after an abrupt change in altitude and are usually worse at night.

Both HAPE and HACE are considered medical emergencies. They can result in serious complications and even death if not promptly recognized and treated. If medical attention is not readily available, you should descend a minimum of 2,000 feet or until the symptoms resolve. Again, those of you who want to venture to altitudes above 12,000 feet need to be prepared to deal with these potential complications by having the appropriate training, equipment, and medication.

Now that we've addressed these basic survival issues, we can talk about how altitude affects performance. One of the first things you'll notice when you exercise at high altitude is that it's harder to catch your breath. Maximal oxygen consumption decreases by approximately 10% for every 3,000 feet above 5,000 feet, which is nearly a mile above sea level. Your aerobic performance will be worse, and you may experience decreased strength and coordination. Your sleep may be disrupted, and you may experience frequent awakenings during your first few nights at altitudes above 5,000 feet. If you want to be at your best, you are going to need to take some time to acclimatize.

The good news is that under most circumstances you can adapt fairly quickly. Within a couple of days of arriving at a higher altitude, you will begin to make significant changes that will improve your exercise tolerance. By ten to twenty days, you will have completed much of your initial adaptation to altitude. Since it may take months to reach near maximal adaptation, you'll need to do some planning if you want to be at your best.

Individuals who have been raised at high altitude seem to have an advantage, and some cultural groups that have lived at extremely high altitudes for generations have an even greater advantage.

Regardless of your background, you'll need to take your time acclimating if you have spent a significant amount of time at sea level. Try to plan a gradual ascent to less than 8,000 feet on your first day. To increase your chances of getting a restful sleep, try to sleep below this level on your first few nights. Many athletes find it helpful to venture to higher altitudes during the day and return to the lower altitudes at night.

As you get accustomed to the thinner air, you can begin to increase your level of exertion remembering that it will take time to adjust. Finally, you have to realize that there is just less air at high altitude, so don't expect to achieve the same level of aerobic performance that you do when you're at sea level.

Chapter 6

Hone Your Skills

Now that you are physically and mentally ready to perform, let's focus on developing the skills that you'll need for your sport. We'll see how developing good technique is one the most important aspects of successful athletic performance.

One of the hardest parts of learning a new skill is staying motivated when you don't seem to be improving. You'll be able to stay motivated if you understand the learning process and how practice helps you to improve your skills. In this chapter we will also see how you can get the most out of your workouts by properly structuring your practice sessions. Finally, there are also some good ideas about feedback and mental practice that are worth knowing about. Like so much of the information in the previous chapters, this information has many applications, so I hope you get a lot out of it.

Let's take a look at a basic motor skill, like pitching a baseball, to point out some of the important aspects of good technique. To simplify matters, let's get the batter out of the batter's box and just focus on speed and accuracy. Try to throw the ball with just your arm. Don't twist your torso and don't step. Not very impressive. Now try it again, but allow yourself to twist your torso and step into the direction of the throw. Much better. Now wind up, lift your leg, and throw the ball as you step forward.

In this example, you substantially improved you ability to throw by simply varying the technique. You could have spent years in the gym doing strength training to achieve the gains in velocity that you just got from changing your technical approach. Improving your technique increases the power and efficiency of an activity by taking advantage of five basic principles.

Preloading involves stretching your muscles to the appropriate length before loading the muscle. This takes all of the slack out of your muscle and allows you to take advantage of the most powerful segment of muscle contraction. Your muscles

96

can contract over a specific range, and the strength of contraction varies with muscle length. At the shortest and longest extremes of muscle length, the force of contraction is weakest. When your muscle length is in the intermediate ranges, you get the strongest contractile force. You do this naturally when you bring your arm back to throw or when you squat down a bit before you jump. Try this out by attempting to jump from your tiptoes without bending your legs. Then try from a slightly squatted position with your feet flat on the ground.

Leverage improves as a result of proper positioning. This is true from two different perspectives. The first has to do with your position in relation to an adjacent object or opponent. One of the major goals of Jiu-Jitsu, for example, is to continually work toward a position that gives you better leverage against an opponent. The second perspective involves stabilizing and positioning body segments so that the most mobile body segment is in the best position to perform the desired activity. Throwing the ball after planting both feet on the ground while your torso begins to face the target is more effective than trying to throw it while you're off balance and facing the wrong direction. Establishing a good base will improve your leverage and is an important part of good technique for many sports.

Momentum can increase the effectiveness of many activities. It frequently involves a coordinated shift in your center of gravity. Jumpers can convert forward momentum into higher and longer jump by getting a running start. Many techniques in sports require some degree of momentum before they can actually be performed. Try to imagine a pole vault without a running start or a discus throw without a windup. Discus throwing, by the way, is a good example of how rotational momentum can help improve the effectiveness of an activity. In some sports, you can use your opponent's momentum to manipulate the situation. Basketball players will fake to get the opponent's momentum to go one way while they quickly slide around in the other direction. Many forms of self-defense use the attacker's momentum to increase the effectiveness of defensive strikes or throws.

Synergy is the coordinated effort of several muscle groups. It's getting every cell in your body to pitch in on the task. Our pitching example shows the importance of leg and torso action when it is combined with arm motion. Every muscle has to fire in a precise sequence to get this effect. Since you can't consciously control each muscle fiber, you'll have to stay loose and let them work together. Staying physically relaxed not only feels good, it can help you practice what you're trying to learn. That is, if you're trying to learn how to develop a fluid pitch, repeating the stiff-man version might not be the best approach.

Timing means doing the right thing, at the right place, and the right time. You can see how timing and synergy are closely related because to get your muscles to work together they have to fire at precisely the right moment. Timing takes on an added dimension in sports that require you to coordinate your motion with rapid changes in your environment. A baseball or fast-pitch softball hitter can have a masterfully coordinated swing, but if he or she is a second late, the ball has already moved out of the zone where they can reap the benefits of preloading, synergy, leverage, and momentum.

Good technique isn't just about improving power and efficiency. A good technical approach can improve accuracy by stabilizing the most dynamic body part so that it is more likely to move in the preferred direction. Our pitching example will serve us well to illustrate this point. If the pitcher takes all the necessary actions to step toward the plate during the pitch, then it is safe to say that the path of least resistance is going to be in the direction of the plate and not center field. From the beginning of the pitch, there are a variety of checkpoints that help keep you pointed in the right direction. They begin with your foot position on the mound, the direction of your initial kick, and your arm position when you're cocking back. They end with the point of release and direction of your follow-through. By maintaining good form throughout the delivery to the follow-through, the pitcher also is able to complete the pitch and be in a good position to field the ball, if necessary.

Each checkpoint positions your body in a way that guides your hand through a course that aligns the most accurate path with the path of least resistance. An archer who has a solid stance and releases the arrow between heartbeats minimizes the likelihood of unwanted movement as she aims for her target. A surfer that is properly balanced on top of his board can respond to the moment-by-moment variations in the immediate environment and position himself in the best part of the wave. Go ahead and take a moment to think about how technique affects accuracy in your sport.

My final point for technique is to show you how using good technique and creating a smooth, fluid motion can help you prevent overuse injuries. By getting your legs, torso, and arms to work together, you'll be using more muscle fibers to do the job. A poorly performed backhand in tennis is notorious for causing an injury known as tennis elbow. It frequently results from trying to muscle the backhand with your wrist and arm. This type of swing not only results in a wimpy shot, it also increases the workload on the muscles around the elbow and forearm.

You can avoid this problem by developing a backhand that utilizes all of the aspects of good technique. This includes bringing the racquet back early (pre-load), establishing a good stance (leverage), shifting your weight from the back leg to the front (momentum), rotating your torso as you shift your weight and swing the racquet (torsional momentum and synergy), and hitting the ball just in front of your body (leverage and timing). The result is a much stronger backhand with less strain on the muscles of the forearm.

Now that I've sold you on the value of good technique, we can start to talk about how you can develop it. The first step is to calm down. It typically takes ten years to become an expert at anything, so relax. The learning process is complicated, but it can be simplified into two basic stages: learning to perform the skill, then learning how to apply the skill to the millions of different situations where that skill is needed (Lee 1991). It may seem overwhelming at first, but you have a variety of tools to help you learn more efficiently. Let's look at what happens during the early, middle, and advanced stages of the leaning process. That way you can get a better understanding about what to focus on during each stage.

Early Stages of Learning

Motivation is one of the key factors during the early phases of learning. Staying motivated is easy if you are having success. It's when you're struggling that frustration sets in, and you start thinking about giving up (Cox 1998). To keep from getting too discouraged, you'll want to remember that early performance is not a great predictor of future performance (Magill 1998, p. 284).

Losing or making an error doesn't have to be a complete loss either. You can learn as much from losing as you can from winning. As a matter of fact, in Jiu-Jitsu we sometimes perform practice drills where we let our opponent beat us. This allows you to see firsthand how they set up the attack and then execute the move. Seeing the move from a completely different perspective gives you an opportunity to explore the different possibilities for defense and counterattacks. This approach keeps you focused on your main goal: learning and having fun and not just winning.

Keeping Score

Winning or losing, scores and statistics are all a particular type of feedback, and this is probably as good a time as any to introduce the concept of feedback and how it plays a role in the learning process. Figure 6.2 (Magill 1998) illustrates the different types of feedback and how they are divided into two main categories: task-intrinsic feedback and augmented feedback.

Task intrinsic feedback: (what you personally sense)

Visual
Auditory (hearing)
Proprioceptive (position)
Tactile (touch)

Augmented feedback: (outside information)

Knowledge of results
Knowledge of performance

Figure 6.2. Different types of feedback related to learning and performing motor skills. (Magillp.186)

Since task-intrinsic feedback and augmented feedback sound like technical mouthfuls, I'm going to refer to task-intrinsic feedback as personal feedback because it is what you'll personally experience when you perform the task. Augmented feedback is feedback that you'll get from outside sources.

You can see from the diagram that personal (task-intrinsic) feedback involves your senses. These include visual, auditory, proprioceptive, and tactile. The first two are fairly self-explanatory. *Proprioceptive feedback* is the sensory information that lets you know where your body parts are in relationship to each other. Thanks to your proprioceptive senses, when you stand up and close your eyes, you still know that you are standing even though you can't see yourself standing. Tactile senses are just another way of saying your sense of touch.

Outside (augmented) feedback is the information that you get from outside your body regarding results and performance. As you can see, these are divided into two types. *Knowledge of results* is the feedback that you get regarding the outcome of a particular action or whether you achieved your goal. The umpire calling a strike and the height mark on the horizontal bar that you just jumped over are examples of external feedback about the result of what you just did.

Knowledge of performance is the outside information about the movement charac-teristics of your performance. These include comments like, "You aren't getting the racquet back in time to hit the ball in front of you," or "I like the way you followed through after hitting that serve." This type of information is directed at trying to augment your sensory input of the performance.

What is so important about feedback?

The problem is that there can be so much feedback, so much to pay attention to, that it becomes difficult to decide what to focus on. Some types of feedback can draw your attention to a less important aspect of your performance and hinder your progress. Let's go out and practice some tennis serves to see how this works. You are going to keep track of whether the serve goes in (knowledge of results). Armed with a bucket of balls and a few tips from your expensive tennis instructor, you stand at the service line to hit a few serves just like the pro showed you. The serve that she demonstrated was a relaxed dynamic serve utilizing a full swing and a dynamic body motion. Unfortunately, the ball is going everywhere except that odd-shaped little box on the other side of the net.

Now that you are zero for ten, you start to get demoralized, and you decide to shorten your swing and stiffen your arm. Look at that, it went in! Let's see if we can repeat that. Two in a row! Now we are starting to get a little motivated. Unfortunately, you are not practicing the serve that you need to be focusing on; instead you're becoming the king of the stiff-man serve. Keeping track of the score changed your entire focus from getting the feel and timing of a smooth, dynamic motion to practicing whatever it takes to get the ball in.

Fortunately, the tennis pro walks by and notices that you are taking the wrong approach. She provides a little outside feedback that improves your knowledge of performance: "What's the matter? You forgot to oil your joints this morning?" She demonstrates a smooth serve and then watches you try a few. This gets you back on track, focused on a new goal, and motivated by the right type of feedback.

Not only is the type of feedback important, so is the frequency. Getting external feedback on every try can be distracting if you are trying to learn a new skill (Weeks 1998). It may be better to limit external feedback to every third or fourth trial so that you can focus your attention on getting the feel of what you're doing.

One of the main benefits of having a coach or trainer is that they can help you stay focused on the right task. Unfortunately, not all coaches are created equally, and you can end up getting a ton of demoralizing, distracting feedback. This is when you want to have an idea of what to focus on so you can filter out useless information and stay on the right track.

In the early stages of learning, the score is not incredibly important. Although keeping score can be motivating under the right circumstances, you may want to pay more attention to getting the feel of performing the skill so that the score doesn't distract you. One way to keep the two processes separate is to take a moment to think about how it felt to perform the task before you turn your attention to the result. We'll come back to this point a little later when we look at practice structure. For the time being, it's better to pay more attention to getting the feel of the game instead of keeping track of the score.

In addition to getting feedback about results, the beginning athlete can also get outside feedback about the performance characteristics of the skill that they are trying to learn. Under the best circumstances, the feedback you get from your coach will help you improve the technical aspects of your performance and keep you motivated. You will also want to be aware of when this type of feedback is distracting and demoralizing so that you can tune it out.

Outside feedback is valuable when it can draw your attention to a specific aspect of performing a skill that helps you to improve your technique. Feedback can be focused on what you are doing correctly or on the mistakes that you are making. Both types of feedback can be helpful in the learning process. Positive feedback is motivating and helps reinforce correct performance. Unfortunately, beginner athletes take the wrong approach, and the only solution is to have someone point out the error. This type of information might remind you to bring your racquet back sooner, step toward the mound, or work on the follow-through. It helps to draw your attention to a part of your performance that will improve your skills if altered in the prescribed way.

The way this information is delivered is also important. By delivering this information in the context of how it relates the entire performance, you can draw your attention to a specific aspect of your performance without interrupting the feel of performing the motion in its entirety. This type of feedback might sound like, "Try to get the feel of how you hit the ball better when you bring your racquet back sooner."

In this example the advice, "bring your racquet back sooner," becomes a part of getting the feel of hitting the ball and not a distraction. Notice how this comment subtly suggests some optimism about your ability to improve your performance. In addition to providing important information in a nondistracting way, it also helps to keep you motivated.

Compare that feedback to: "How many times do I have to tell you to bring your racquet back?" Not only is this statement insulting and demoralizing, it also focuses your attention on just one mechanical aspect of your swing.

Maybe this is a good time to take a brief reality break. You're probably thinking that this is pretty good information, but what control do you have over the kind of feedback that your coach gives you? You might as well try to manipulate the stock market with the $25 in your piggy bank. Some coaches already know everything anyway, that's why they are the coaches, and you are the student.

Let's see what options you have. One is to buy them a copy of this book for their birthday. I really like this idea because it will increase my book sales, but it may take them until all the cows have come home to get to this point in the book. A better idea might be to translate what your coach is saying into something that is more effective. Recall from the first chapter that you can learn to tune out the less useful information and look for any valuable part of the message. You can build on this by taking whatever useful information your coach is trying to tell you and create a new statement that integrates the useful information into the overall scheme of what you are trying to learn. Think back on some of those wonderful comments from your well-intentioned coaches, and see if you can come up with some healthier thoughts to bounce around inside your head.

"The reason you can't hit the side the of barn with your fastball is that your front foot is landing all over the place." It really means: "Get the feel of how stepping toward the plate improves your accuracy."

"Your serve is awful." Translate that to: "Let's see what we can do to improve your serve."

The important point is to prevent the negative commentary from bouncing around in your head by replacing it with thoughts that help you stay motivated and improve your performance. Turning a negative comment into something positive is just another opportunity to practice staying cool in the face of aggression. You might want to go back and review some of the suggestions for handling obnoxious people from the first chapter. Learning this skill will not only be helpful in sports but will be valuable in many other aspects of your life.

Traditionally, athletes have gotten feedback in the form of verbal communication or direct demonstration of a specific skill by a coach or instructor. With the help of technology, athletes can now get feedback from a variety of electronic gadgets including videotape, force transducers (devices to measure force applied during an activity), electronic muscle sensors, and velocity sensors. This type of feedback is valuable as your skills improve, and you move into the advanced stages of learning.

Besides getting feedback, there are a few things you can do to make the learning process a little easier. They involve breaking the movement into parts or simplifying some aspect of the activity. If an activity is relatively complex, it may be helpful to get oriented to the parts before you work on the entire move. A gymnast might decide to work on one segment of a long routine before she goes on to learn the next segment. This approach is more effective if the parts are not highly interdependent. On the other hand, some routines are difficult to break up because they require a certain degree of momentum and timing. You can practice the approach to a long jump by itself, but when it comes to practicing the jump, you have to do the approach to get the momentum you need to perform the jump.

Another way to simplify is to slow down some aspect of the activity. You can practice "block, punch, and kick" slowly several times, and then gradually increase the speed as you start to feel more comfortable with the transitions from one move to the next. If your sport involves a rapidly moving object, like a baseball going 90 mph, you can practice hitting a ball that is moving slowly at first. When you are the one that is moving, such as in skiing, you can keep your speed down by staying on slopes that are not as steep. Surfers can start in surf that is small then gradually take on bigger surf as they become more confident.

Equipment can also have an effect on the complexity and difficulty of a sport. Beginners can choose equipment that is a little less responsive and more forgiving to help them get the basics of the technique. Once they have the basics down, then they can start transferring those skills to high-performance equipment.

I always had difficulty skiing in crud, a condition in which a heavy layer of snow is covered with a thin layer of ice that can't sustain the weight of skis. It was a major source of frustration to be cruising along the groomed slope like a pro then get instantaneously demoted to a beginner because I hit a patch of thick, crusted-over crud. Then one day, I tried a pair of skis that were designed for skiing in this type of snow and bang! The light went on. Unfortunately, skiing on this type of ski was like driving down the mountain in an old Cadillac, and what I really wanted was something more responsive. I put on a pair of high-performance skis and went out looking for some crud. No problem! Now that I knew what to do, I was able to transfer my newly learned skills to the high-performance skis. The moral of the story is that the right type of equipment can help you make breakthroughs in areas that you are having difficulty with.

Intermediate and Advanced Stages of Learning

Now that you have some basic skills at your command, you are ready to move on to the intermediate stages of learning. As you recall, there are two basic stages to learning a motor skill: learning the basic movements and then learning to apply those movements in a variety of settings, also called *parameterization*. Learning a basic backhand is one thing, but making a decision about what side the ball is coming to, at what velocity, with how much top spin, and how it might bounce up from the court is a completely different endeavor.

As you transition to the intermediate stages of learning, your ability to apply the basic skills you've learned to each situation will be as important as performing the skill itself. Sometimes it seems impossible to react quickly when presented with so many potential variables. A major league baseball hitter has 1/3 of a second to come up with a decision about what to do with a 3½-inch, 90-mph problem every time he goes up to bat.

Fortunately, God has equipped you with an incredible piece of equipment: a nervous system. Within a fraction of a second, a skilled athlete is capable of making an accurate assessment of a unique problem and almost simultaneously they are able to execute an equally precise solution. Although it can take a number of approaches to improve your ability, I would like to focus on three main topics: strategy, focus, and practice.

Strategy

As you begin to understand the strategies in your sport, you'll be able to get a jump on your opponent by narrowing the possibilities for the next move. For example, with a base runner on first, the catcher has to look for the runner to steal, and the second baseman has to be ready to get to the ball and tag the runner. Any hesitation to think about what happens next will place the defense at a disadvantage. In football, if it's third down and fifteen yards, the defense is going to be aware of the high probability of a pass, but if it is third down and inches, they're going to be looking for a run. These are basic examples of how understanding strategy can give you a definite advantage. Your job is to become a proficient mind reader by learning the tactics your opponents will use.

After training in Jiu-Jitsu for several years, I had the privilege to train with Helio Gracie, the founder of Gracie Jiu-Jitsu. At that time, he was eighty-five years young and was weighing 132 pounds. After easily defending every attack I could muster, he began to throw in a few attacks of his own. Within a few seconds, he would start to chuckle, and I would quickly become aware that I was within millimeters of defeat. He would then ease up and start to formulate a completely new attack. I would try to defend and within a few seconds he would start to chuckle again. I felt just enough discomfort to know that I was trapped again. Over and over he would attack; I would defend or try to counterattack, and he would reposition and attack again. Sooner rather than later, I was cooked.

Finally, he let me stop to catch my breath and regain my composure. He said, "Doctor, you are much younger and stronger than I am; you know almost all the same moves that I know. As a matter of fact, you know every move that I used to defeat you. The main advantage that allows me to beat you so easily is not that I know more techniques than you do or that I can perform each technique much better than you can. It is because I know what you are going to do before you know what you are going to do." With every move I made, not only did he have a response, but he also had already narrowed the possibilities for how I would react. He had his next action plan ready before I even began to move. At each juncture, he systematically narrowed my options and before I knew it, I was trapped.

He went on to say that practicing Jiu-Jitsu is like playing chess with your body; it's primarily a game of staying one or two moves ahead of your opponent. Whether you are a golfer trying to hit the ball in a crosswind or a basketball player playing his opponent a little to the right, having a good strategy and being able to anticipate the next move will give you an important advantage.

Focus

Once you have a good understanding of the strategies in your sport, you'll know where to direct your focus. This means knowing how to direct your attention to the earliest and most reliable clue of the next play. Again, with a man on first base, the catcher is not just focusing on his usual duties of catching the ball. He is watching the guy on first out of the corner of his eye for the first hint that he's going for second base. The second baseman is also looking for the guy on first to move, as is the center fielder that will need to back up the second baseman if the catcher makes a bad throw. Everyone involved is anticipating the next move and directing their attention appropriately.

One of the goals of the intermediate-level athlete is to learn how to focus their attention on the aspect of their environment that will give them the earliest and most reliable clue as to what is going to happen next.

A basketball player on defense might want to focus on her opponent's upper abdomen as she begins to drive toward the basket because it is the most reliable indicator of which way she is really going to go. If she is watching her opponent's eyes and head, the offensive player can do a quick head fake in one direction, move in the opposite direction, and be a fraction of a second ahead of the defense.

A baseball hitter wants to increase his chances of making contact by focusing on the ball from the anticipated point of delivery. A soccer player charging down the field not only has to pay attention to the ball but also to what the defense is doing. I'd like to go on and on with examples, but every sport is full of pivotal situations that help you to predict the next play. A good coach can help you improve by showing you where to direct your attention.

Practice

The third way to improve your performance is to practice. There's no way around it. You can read, watch the pros, and learn the strategies, but there's no substitute for getting in there and trying it over and over. Hence the old adage, "Practice makes perfect." Green Bay Packers coaching legend Vince Lombardi took it even further when he said, "Perfect practice makes perfect." The main question is whether there is a better way to practice. Is there an approach that results in a quicker development of good technique and improved performance? To answer these questions, we will want to look at how practice results in learning and review the advantages and disadvantages of the different approaches to practice.

One of the key aspects of practice is repetition. Initially, it may appear that the result of repetition is memorization and, in fact, some of the basic characteristics of a given activity do require some degree of memorization. These basic characteristics are called the invariant characteristics of a motor pattern (Schmidt 1975, 2003). Okay, that sounds reasonable, but if all of our responses are memorized, what happens when we are faced with a novel situation? The experienced athlete is able to create an effective response to each new challenge. In fact, every sports situation is truly unique. Every pitch is different, every wave is unique, and each serve is one of a kind. That's part of the fun and challenge of being involved in sports.

As we mentioned before, the process of applying your basic motor skills to unique situations is called parameterization. This involves assessing the situation while quickly preparing and executing a response. Everything that happens in your mind before you move is known as the cognitive or premotor phase. Ideally, your practice should be structured in a way that promotes both the cognitive phase of learning as well as motion phase.

The question now becomes how do you structure your practice to maximize both the cognitive *and* physical aspects of the activity that you are trying to improve? To answer this question we'll want to take a look at what happens with repetition. Let's go back out to the tennis court and work on our backhand with the tennis ball machine. After the first few tries, you've gotten the feel of where the ball is going to bounce and how you're going to approach it. Since the ball is coming at you the same way each time, you've eliminated a great deal of variability and simplified the cognitive part of your practice. After a while, the tendency is to completely ignore the cognitive phase and just become a robot that returns the ball to the other side of the net. You can start thinking about tonight's date or tomorrow's meeting while your body works away at that backhand.

The confusing part about practicing this way is that while you are practicing, your performance will improve. From the surface it may appear as though this might be the best way to learn. Fortunately, it is not; it would make your practice boring. Although your performance improves during this type of practice, when you go test yourself in a random situation, your performance is not as good as the person who includes variability in their practice (Shea 1990; Wrisberg 1991; Bortoli 1992). Variable practice works better because under random conditions you practice solving the problem as well as performing the motor task. In most sports, the premotor component is just as important as performing the motor task itself.

To get the most out of your practice, you'll want to make it as close to the real thing as possible by including a substantial amount of variability and randomness. This approach will ensure that you are practicing the cognitive aspect of your sport as well as the basic motor skill.

Before you get carried away with variability, you need to keep in mind that there is a fine balance between how much time you spend focusing on a specific skill and how much variety to include. I can't give you a precise formula for exactly how much variability to include because it changes with your level of expertise and the complexity of your sport. Beginners may want to limit their exposure to variability in an effort to develop some basic skills before they go on to challenge their skills on the playing field. Intermediate-level athletes can begin to add more variety, and advanced athletes should be striving to include as much variety as possible.

Now that we know variety is good, we can talk about how to make it happen. We've already touched on one of the ways to improve variability: avoid mindless repetition. I've been using the terms variability and randomness in a general sense but they have a specific meaning and purpose when you are structuring your practice. The first step in avoiding mindless repetition is to vary the characteristics of a given motion. That is, you can work on your backhand but practice going deep, shallow, across the court, and so on. Once you've developed a sense of confidence in your basic skills you can add randomness by randomly alternating the different skills that you need for your sport. Instead of doing twenty serves in a row, then twenty backhands, and so on, you can practice a couple of serves, switch to backhand, then forehand, and finally volleys. Then you can rotate deep, shallow, and crosscourt for each skill.

After a few rounds, you can take randomness a step further by adding the element of surprise. Your training partner or coach can randomly set up the shots that you need to work on. This will increase your level of alertness and make your practice as realistic as possible.

Another way to increase variety is to change your practice setting. You can do this by changing sides, moving to another court, or changing partners. If you have the option of practicing in a variety of settings, you may want to alternate practice locations throughout the week.

Finally, you'll want to practice in a gamelike setting. The first step is to have a little game just like you would in competition. Try to make it just like the real thing, but don't let the score keep you from practicing what you want to practice. You can step up to lifelike competition by entering small tournaments with comparably skilled athletes. Your goal is to get enough experience so that you become comfortable with the pressure and intensity of the competitive setting. To help increase variety in your practice, look at your entire week's practice sessions and try to break them up as much as possible. Avoid focusing a single session on one specific skill; instead, try to spread practicing that skill over several sessions during the week. Also, during a specific practice session, try not to repeat the same exact technique over and over. Try taking turns after a couple of tries, switching sides, changing training partners, or moving to a different area.

I'd like to clarify one thing at this point. There are situations when it is extremely valuable for intermediate and advanced athletes to focus on a particular aspect of their sport. During certain phases of learning, performance plateaus frustrate some athletes. They get stuck at a certain level because they are having difficulty performing a technically complex task. This can be quite a problem if it is a pivotal aspect of your sport. A tennis player may be having trouble with their backhand or a pitcher with their curveball. Under these circumstances, it will be refreshing to spend a little extra time focusing on the problematic area by thoroughly dissecting every step and making sure that you are using the best technical approach.

You can still maintain a healthy degree of variety by exploring all the different variations that may be associated with that activity. You can focus on your backhand, but still mix it up by trying to practice returning a backhand that is coming at you short, deep, fast, slow, crosscourt, or down the line. You can practice your transition from a forehand shot to a backhand shot or from a serve to a backhand shot. This allows you to include other aspects of your sport while practicing the dynamics of setting up and executing your backhand. You can also add variety to your backhand workout by practicing it with different partners or on different sides of the court.

The point that I am trying to make here is to avoid doing the same drill over and over. Try to sneak in some practice on your other skills by adding some dynamic transitions to and from the skill that you are trying to focus on.

Mental Practice

Now that we've established the importance of the cognitive phase of practice, it will be easy to see how mental practice will improve your performance. Although mental practice is a distinct mental process, it utilizes many of the same mental processes that you use to prepare and execute a motor skill (Stephan 1996). By alternating mental practice with actual practice, you'll get better results than if you just rest between tries (Kohl 1992). Whether you are tired, injured, or just waiting for your next turn, you can continue to improve your skills by mentally practicing what you're trying to learn (Ahern 1997).

One way to practice is just to watch other people perform what you are trying to learn. You can increase the effectiveness of watching by becoming an active participant. Go ahead and place yourself in the position of the skilled athlete. See and feel everything as though you were the one that was in his position. Try to position yourself in a way that allows you to see what's coming at you and then mimic his motion and timing. This can be incredibly helpful in complicated skills where timing and momentum are crucial.

Cross-country skiing is a good example of how you can spend hours hearing about how to put your hand in this position, pole over here, and slide your ski forward only to find yourself tied up in a knot at the bottom of the hill. You can get a quick boost by simply watching a skilled athlete and rehearsing the activity in your mind before you actually try to perform it. This tool works even if the person that you are watching is not an expert (McCullagh 1997). Once you have the basic timing, you can focus on getting the feel of adapting your technique to the moment-by-moment changes in terrain and snow conditions.

There are a variety of ways that you can use mental practice to improve your skills (White 1996). One way is to watch yourself performing the task as though you were an observer. This approach is called *external visual imagery* and it involves trying to create an external vision or model of what you're going to be doing. It's like looking at a picture or watching a video of your performance. This approach is most effective when the form of an activity is important. It has valuable applications in sports where a fixed position or pose is part of the performance, but it also has applications in dynamic situations.

In contrast to external visual imagery is *internal visual imagery*. This approach is particularly helpful when trying to maneuver through an environment like a race-course. It's also useful when you need to be able to focus on certain visual cues like a target, an approaching ball, or an opponent. Being able to visualize and focus on important visual cues can help with the premotor portion of your activity and prepare you for the next type of imagery: *kinesthetic imagery*. When you perform this type of mental practice, you are trying to feel what it's like to perform the task. This type of imagery is particularly useful in complex motor tasks like diving and gymnastics.

Let's use hitting a baseball to illustrate how to use each type of mental practice. Go ahead, step into the batter's box, and get ready to hit some balls. As you prepare for the pitch, you have a mental image of what a hitter's stance is going to look like, so you try to conform to this image. Your feet are in a specific position, your knees are slightly bent, and your hands are back. You may switch your attention to how it feels to be in that position by becoming aware of your grip on the bat and how your weight is distributed.

Now that you are ready, you can focus your attention on the pitcher. You can see him standing on the mound getting ready to start his windup. As he begins the pitch, you focus your attention on the area where his arm is going to appear just prior to the release of the ball. You can see his arm coming straight over, and you begin to track the ball during its approach. It's a fastball coming right down the middle; you continue to track the ball as you shift your attention to how it's going to feel to begin your swing. The bat comes around, and you feel it collide with the ball in the sweetest part of the swing.

You can replay the pitch in slow motion, frame by frame, or real time. You can change the pitch so that you can get used to picking up the curveballs and adjust your swing appropriately. Put in a right-handed pitcher then a lefty. You're in control right now, so explore all the possibilities. Just be sure that you are in a safe environment and not in a situation where you should be paying attention to something else.

There are a couple of other points that I want to make about mental practice. First, one of the ways that mental practice can help you is by decreasing performance anxiety (Halvari 1996). The other point has to do with rehearsing your mental state while you are doing your mental practice. Remember how we talked about the importance of your mental state during chapter one? Well, performing at your best means being in that ideal performance state or being "in the zone." It's that state of mind where there's an optimal mix of excitement and relaxation. It's no surprise that it is easier to learn while you are in this state of mind because timing and synergy work better when you are relaxed. You can practice getting to this state of mind in just about any setting. You can practice dealing with anxiety-provoking situations, catcalls, and harassment by mentally placing yourself in those types of situations and then experiencing how you maintain the ideal state of mind during your performance.

Getting in this relaxed, playful state is important for effective learning because it allows you to take some chances and explore different possibilities much like a child would experience playing on the playground. This is the spirit that you need when you are trying to learn a new skill. After all, what you are trying to do is to learn how to play.

CHAPTER 7

Optimal Training

It can get pretty dull if your sport becomes all work and no play. What used to be fun becomes daily suffering, and as you push your body to the limit, you'll find that it gets harder and harder to recover. Your performance begins to drop off. Maybe it's because you're not trying hard enough, so you redouble your efforts only to find that you're going nowhere. You feel tired but you're not sleeping well. Your friends haven't told you how irritable you are because they are afraid you might rip their arms off. Finally, you decide to take a day off. You feel a little better, but you're still not all there.

To perform at your best, you are going to need to push extremely hard at times, and the harder you push yourself, the greater the risk that you'll end up overtraining. Your challenge is to be able to tell when enough is enough.

In this chapter, we'll see what can happen if you continually overdo it. You'll learn to recognize the earliest signs of overtraining and how to design a training program that results in maximal performance with minimal risk.

Overtraining

The most common symptoms of overtraining are fatigue, decreased performance, and chronic muscle pain. Well, every self-respecting athlete has some pain or fatigue, and everyone is a little off the mark at times. It's when you fail to recognize the signs and continue to push that the problems begin. You don't want to make this mistake because once you become overtrained it may take weeks or even months to recover (Fry 1997). Table 7.1 lists some of the major signs of overtraining.

The following are symptoms of overtraining:

- Fatigue
- Decreased performance
- Weight loss
- Increased resting heart rate*
- Decreased appetite
- Depression
- Sleep difficulty
- Irritability
- Frequent illness
- Injury
- Weakness
- Mood changes

*Increased heart rate may be an early, transient finding.

Table 7.1. Signs of overtraining.

The physiology of overtraining is still somewhat of a mystery. Exercise scientists have identified a number of chemical and hormonal abnormalities in athletes who overtrain. In the early stages of overtraining, chronic elevations of adrenaline will increase your resting heart rate, make you irritable, and upset your normal sleep patterns. If you continue to overtrain, a different set of hormones appear and the result is a lower heart rate, both at rest and during exercise (Kenetta 1998).

Lower testosterone levels combined with increasing cortisol levels can be an indication that your body is moving from a state of building itself up to a state of chronic breakdown (Urhausen 1995). There are even changes in your immune system that can make it harder for you to fight off infection (Mackinnon 1997).

In addition to hormonal and immunological markers, sports scientists are also monitoring lactic acid levels (Fry 1997; Snyder 1993) and plasma viscosity (Benhaddad 1999) as indicators of overtraining. Lactic acid accumulates with muscle exhaustion, and plasma viscosity can be used as a marker to diagnose muscle fatigue or severe cramping. I'm sure that in the future we'll be seeing more sophisticated ways of monitoring highly competitive athletes, but the signs in Table 7.1 will do a good job of letting you know when it's time to back off.

One way that athletes improve their level of conditioning is to plan relatively short periods of heavy training or overreaching. If you are going to use this approach, you'll need to closely monitor yourself for signs of overtraining, and be sure to plan plenty of time for rest and recovery.

There is no precise formula for how hard and how long you can push before you have to drop back. It depends on your level of conditioning and where you are in your training cycle. External factors such as illness, injury, and even the amount of day-to-day stress in your life can have an effect on how much physical stress you can endure (Kentta 1998).

The best advice that I can find is to try to limit your overreaching cycles to less than three weeks. Try to alternate hard days with easy days and take one full day off per week (Lehmann 1997). Listen to your body. If you start to experience ritualistic, daily pain plus fatigue and your performance starts to drop off, then you'll know that it's time for a break. You should be able to recover from a properly planned overreaching cycle within seventy-two hours (Kentta 1998). You'll know that you've fully recovered if you have none of the signs and symptoms listed in Table 7.1. Once you've established that you're able to recover, you can continue with a moderate to aggressive training program. On the other hand, if you're still dragging after seventy-two hours, you'll want to decrease your training load until you feel fully rested.

Since there's such a fine line between overreaching and overtraining, it's not surprising to see that some athletes have overdone it. If you're starting to drag and can't shake it off with a couple of days of rest, then you'll need to figure out what's wrong before you do more harm. The first step is to visit your family physician to make sure that you don't have some underlying illness that's making you feel so tired. They'll want to review your history, perform a thorough physical exam, and run some basic lab tests. If your physician is familiar with sports medicine, they might review your training program to help you evaluate your overall training load (Derman 1997). Once they have ruled out an illness, you can get started on your road to recovery.

There are a variety of rejuvenation strategies with common theme of rest, nutrition, and stress management. Athletes with severe fatigue may need to cut their training programs to the bare minimum to get started. One approach is to begin with divided sessions of low intensity aerobic activity lasting five to ten minutes per day. Try to keep your heart rate between 120 and 140 beats per minute during this phase. You can gradually increase the duration of your workouts so that you're up to an hour within six to twelve weeks.

Once you've established a good endurance base, you can start to increase your intensity by adding ten second intervals of high intensity training separated by three to five minutes of recovery. Be sure to fully recover from your intense workouts and take at least one full day off every week. Decreasing your training load works so well that many athletes are pleasantly surprised at how well they are performing after twelve weeks of relatively low intensity training (Budgett 1998).

You're probably thinking that taking twelve weeks to recover sounds like a lot of lost time. It is. That's why an ounce of prevention is worth a pound of cure. You can decrease the chances of overdoing it by attending to the details of good nutrition and hydration during any of your overreaching cycles. You can balance your heavy training load by allowing yourself enough time to get a little extra sleep, take a nap, stretch, or get a massage.

Before

1. Prehydration: stay hydrated during the day and drink 400 to 600 ml of fluid two hours before practice and then 200 ml right before the start of practice.
2. Nutrition: attend to good nutrition throughout the day then have about 300 grams (2 g/lb of body weight) of complex carbohydrate four hours before and 150 g (1/2 g/lb of body weight) one hour before exercise.
3. Rest: plan 20 to 30 min a day of R&R during periods of heavy exertion.
4. Stress management: avoid taking on extra projects during periods of heavy exertion.
5. Leave time for warm-up and stretching before your workouts.

During

1. Stay hydrated: drink 150–200 ml of sports drink or water every fifteen to twenty minutes. Try to limit fluid losses to less than 2% of body weight.
2. Nutrition: during prolonged exercise, take about 150 g of carbohydrate every hour by using a sports drink, sports bar, bananas, dried fruit, bagels, or your favorite workout snack.

3. Stay cool: take advantage of every available cooling mechanism (i.e., clothing, shade, fans, and fluids).

4. Pace yourself: monitor your heart rate and other signs of exertion.

5. Learn to recover during every break in the action.

6. Stay loose, relax, and have fun.

After

1. Rehydrate: try to get back to your baseline weight within a couple of hours after your workout. Use a sports drink to rehydrate if you lost more than 2% of your body weight during exercise.

2. Nutrition: begin replenishing your carbohydrate stores immediately after your workout.

3. Recover: take full advantage of your favorite recovery mechanisms especially massage, good food, rest, and sleep.

Concerns for Women

Some female athletes undergo a particular type of imbalance between stress and recovery. It's called the *Female Athletic Triad* because they develop disordered eating, loss of their period (amenorrhea), and osteoporosis (Ireland 2004). This is a complex disorder with a strong emotional component. Women who are affected with this problem frequently have a distorted body image and believe that they are fat when they are actually very thin. They become so preoccupied with their appearance that they start to use laxatives or they self-induce vomiting in a desperate attempt to control their weight. Other women with this problem will train incessantly to keep their weight down.

One of the toughest aspects of treating athletes with this condition is that they are frequently convinced that low body weight improves performance. Unfortunately, the end result of consuming suboptimal calories and nutrients is actually decreased performance, loss of motivation, and injury.

Having a negative caloric balance will disrupt a woman's hormonal cycles, and they'll develop irregular periods or stop menstruating altogether (Manore 1999). For women, estrogen also plays an important role in maintaining strong bones. Without estrogen and calcium a woman's bones become weak and the risk of fracture increases. To make matters worse, having calcium-deficient bones during your late teens and early adulthood can result in weaker bones for your entire life.

Since this condition results in so many long-term physical and emotional problems, it is important to identify high-risk women during the early stages of the illness. Although the Female Athletic Triad can affect athletes in any sport, it is more common in sports where image and body mass are a factor. These include gymnastics, dancing, skating, and long-distance running. The successful treatment of this problem requires appropriate medical and psychological help as well as cooperation and support from friends, family, coaches, and trainers (Putukian 1998).

Not all women who stop having their periods have the Female Athletic Triad. Heavy training loads combined with low caloric intake will frequently result in loss of a period. The difference is the intent. Some women start training harder and get too busy to eat properly. They aren't preoccupied by their weight, but the continual negative caloric balance eventually disrupts their normal hormone cycles. One of the first signs that you are in a negative balance can be that your periods become irregular, and if the same conditions persist, your periods will stop entirely.

Some women welcome the thought of not having periods, but prolonged negative caloric balance can have an adverse effect on your health and performance. Regardless of the intent, if your periods stop, you will still face the same issues regarding missing the opportunity to build peak bone mineral density and have a higher risk of fractures. Most female athletes can regain normal menstrual cycles by establishing a positive or neutral caloric balance, but some athletes may also need to decrease their training loads to get their periods back.

There are a few more points that you might want to know about menstrual cycles in female athletes. Sometimes losing your period can be due to medical problems involving your thyroid gland, pituitary gland, or other major organ systems. It is a good idea to get a checkup if you are not having periods.

Symptoms of Female Athletic Triad include:

- Weight loss
- Difficulty losing weight
- Loss of lean body mass
- Decreased performance
- Fatigue
- Persistent injuries
- Stress fracture
- Slow healing
- Decreased motivation
- Irritability
- Depression
- Poor concentration
- Anemia
- Irregular periods
- No periods
- Frequent illness

Table 7. Negative Caloric Balance. You may be wondering how a negative caloric balance prevents weight loss. Without adequate calories many athletes become fatigued and aren't able to exercise long enough to burn fat (Grandjean 1999).

Another major cause of a missed period is pregnancy. This might seem to be an obvious cause of a missed period, but in some cases denial can be incredibly powerful. Somehow it happens, and it is important to know early so that you can take all the proper precautions. These include seeing an obstetrician, taking prenatal vitamins, and avoiding aspirin, alcohol, and excessive heat. Incidentally, if you are sexually active and think there is even a remote chance that you might get pregnant, you should take prenatal vitamins before you get pregnant.

Some female athletes (and their partners) are surprised to find out that they can get pregnant even though they aren't having periods. Unfortunately, ovulation occurs before menstruation, so a woman can go several months without a period before they ovulate. You can get pregnant if you are sexually active at the time of ovulation. If you are going to be sexually active but aren't ready to start a family, then it is important for you have a good understanding of birth control. Because losing your period due to excessive exercise is a poor birth control method, you'll want to talk to your family physician about better alternatives.

Burnout

You'll know that you're starting to burn out when it no longer feels like it's worth it. There will be the physical symptoms of pain and fatigue, but the final blow is to the head. It's mental. Whatever it was that was driving you is no longer there. If there are any positives, they are crushed by the weight of the negatives. For some athletes, even the thought of participation becomes so painful that they just have to get away from their sport for a while. Many never make it back.

It's not clear why some athletes burn out and others don't. Clearly expectations play a role. If you expect to be a champion and your performance is not of champion caliber, then the regular frustration becomes overwhelming. Your chances of burnout are also greater when you are doing a lot of high volume, monotonous training as opposed to frequent, high intensity training (Lehmann 1997). Finally, psychological intensity can play a role in the athlete who becomes obsessed with their sport. If they are not practicing or playing, then they are thinking or talking about it. It eventually consumes the athlete to the point that he just gets sick of it.

Everyone reaches a point where he wants to decrease his involvement in a sport, and there is nothing the matter with making the transition if you need to. Ideally the transition will occur at a time that suits you.

You can decrease your chances of premature burnout by developing a long-term perspective and having a well-designed training program. In addition to minimizing burnout and injuries, a good training program will also keep you performing at your best.

I've already introduced the concept of periodization as it applies to aerobic conditioning and strength training. Let's take a closer look at how to set up a year-round plan for your training program.

As we already discussed, the way to prevent overtraining is relatively simple: balance your training load and your recovery time. This works so well that most successful athletes include regularly scheduled recovery periods into their workout program. They will preemptively alternate easy days with hard days and sprinkle in some days off when they need to. We've already established that prevention is always better than burnout, and in this case prevention involves both planning and flexibility.

Smarter athletes plan their training programs around two kinds of cycles: macrocycles and microcycles. Macrocycles are the way you vary your training intensity over a long time. You might want to sit down and identify your goals for the year so you can plan your program around your priorities.

Realistically, you can only peak a few times a year. Alternatively, if you have to be at your best for a long season, you may want to limit your peak to once a year. You'll want to be peaking during the most important part of your competitive cycle. A typical cycle involves relative rest, basic conditioning, gradual increased volume and intensity, high intensity practice, tapering, competition, and finally, rest again.

There is no doubt that you need to exercise to improve performance. On the other hand, too much exercise will make you tired and eventually your performance will start to deteriorate. The good news is that as long as you don't overtrain, the training effect of exercise will last longer than the fatigue. If you taper your workouts, your fatigue will begin to diminish, and you'll start to see signs of improved performance. Unfortunately, if you rest too long you will start to lose some of the beneficial effects of your hard work. The challenge facing most athletes is to balance the stress of exercise with the optimal amount of recovery.

Exercise scientists have used information about the effects of training and rest to model an ideal training program. One model suggests that athletes should increase their training intensity but only on alternate days for a season that lasts approximately five months. The intensity of your training should take a triangular profile, concentrating the heaviest training during week twelve through week four before competition. Your hardest week would be approximately six weeks before competition (Morton 1997).

As you get closer to competing, you'll want to *taper* your workouts to take advantage of the beneficial effects of rest. This is when you're going to need to do a little balancing act because if you train too hard, you won't be rested, but if you rest too long, you'll start to get out of shape. Heavy training volumes during the last seven to ten days before competition will have a negative effect on both strength (Gibala 1994) and aerobic (Zarkadas 1995) performance. On the other hand, if you maintain intensity but decrease your overall training volume, you'll see an improvement in performance over the next four to twenty-eight days (Mujica 1998). You may want to set a goal to gradually decrease your training volume by 50%, including a couple of full rest days during the week before competition.

Gradual decreases in training load appear to work better than abrupt changes (Gibala 1994, Zarkadas 1995, Mujica 1998). During your taper, you'll want to keep your intensity at about 70% of your maximal training intensity (Zarkadas 1995). You can monitor the intensity of your workouts subjectively or by using a heart rate monitor.

This program assumes that the athlete is focused on an individual event or a short series of events. What if your competitive season lasts for months?

Let's use a high school basketball player to illustrate this point. Basketball has a relatively long season and Pat, our budding basketball star, has decided that he wants to be at his best during this year's high school season. There will be about eight weeks of intense preseason practice followed by four months of competition. Pat doesn't want to show up for preseason practice out of shape, and he figures that it might take a month and a half to ramp up from his basic conditioning level to his preseason fitness level. Basic fitness might take two months. So far, his program looks like this:

June	July	Aug	Sep	Oct	Nov	Dec	Jan	Feb
Basic training		Ramp up	Preseason practice		Competition			

Let's take a closer look at what is going to happen during each phase of training.

During basic training, Pat is going to focus on improving both his strength and level of aerobic conditioning. He's also going to make it as fun as possible by running at the beach, hiking in the mountains, swimming in the pool, and going to the gym with his friends. Hard days will be followed by easy days, and there will be a minimum of two full days off per week. Pat's going to allow himself the flexibility to go hard if he feels up to it and back off if he doesn't. He is still going to be shooting some baskets and playing some pickup games, but it's all going to be fairly light and completely under his control.

As August starts to roll around, Pat is going to gradually increase the length and intensity of his aerobic workouts. The track is a good place to monitor your pace, so he is going to go there once a week to do some short interval workouts. Once a week he may go for a longer run at an easy pace.

During this phase, he is also going to keep up his strength training, but there is no need to increase the weight because he is focused on developing dynamic strength and not maximal strength. Pat's also going to ask his trainer about some exercises to improve his jumping skills. Throughout this period, he will continue to maintain the same microcycles of alternate hard days and easy days with two full days off per week.

Pat had better be in pretty good shape when preseason practice starts because this is when the coach is going to start to turn up the heat. During this phase of his training cycle, Pat can expect to do some of his toughest workouts to be sure that he is ready for the demands of competitive basketball.

By the time the season starts, Pat will be at his top level of conditioning, and he is going to need to stay in top shape for the next few months. The hardest workouts during the season will be during his games so Pat's coach will plan the practice sessions in a way that focuses on skills and allows for some physical rest on the days immediately before and after the games.

When planning a heavy workout, the coach will need to consider how the fatigue from that workout will affect the team's performance during upcoming competitions. During a busy season when competitive events are coming at you once or twice a week, it makes little sense to exhaust the athletes with long, intense practice sessions because it may take over a week to fully recover. The goal for the competitive season is to maintain peak conditioning by focusing on shorter intense practice balanced with adequate rest. The stress of performing long, hard workouts is best suited for preseason conditioning.

Pat's training program takes up nine months of the year. During the remaining three months, Pat isn't going to lie around and eat French fries. He may want to get involved in a structured basketball program for part of this time. The difference will be in his attitude. He will rest more often and back off at the first sign of an injury. Whatever he does during this time period will be in a low-pressure environment that will allow him to maintain some basic fitness and develop the skills he needs to be a better basketball player.

Avoid Common Injuries

If you continue to push yourself beyond the limit, your body will start to break down. It's frequently the carelessness that comes with exhaustion that places the final straw on your overstressed body. The end result is a strain or a fracture. For many athletes this is enough to slow them down and rightfully so. Unfortunately, some athletes have trouble getting the message, and they continue to fight on only to find that they have seriously injured themselves. Some of the injuries last for the rest of the season; others are permanent.

Let me just say that medical science has come a long way, but there is really nothing as good as the original equipment. Replacement parts for humans are hard to come by, and they usually don't work very well. Your best bet is to take good care of your body so that you can continue to use it later.

Injuries can be divided into two different types: acute and chronic. Acute injuries seem to happen all at once. You might miss a step and sprain your ankle. There is not much that you can do at this point. You have to treat the injury, and do your best to stay in shape until you are completely recovered. Some athletes try to return before they are ready only to reinjure themselves. They find themselves back at square one or worse: they've done more serious damage.

Trust me, this is not the position that you want to be in. An acute injury implies that some part of your body has been significantly damaged or weakened. To increase your chances of complete recovery, you have to do it right the first time. This is why having a basic understanding of some common injuries will help you develop a better sense of respect for the recovery process.

Fractures

A fracture occurs when a sudden force breaks the integrity of a bone. The results can range from a clean break to an explosion with multiple pieces of bone pointed in every direction. Fractures become more complicated when they involve the joint surface or a child's growth plate, part of a bone where growth occurs. Growth plates are more vulnerable to injury than other parts of the bone. The treatment of most fractures requires realignment of the bones and some method of stabilization. In simple cases, doctors can externally realign the bone and apply a cast to hold the bone in the best position. In more complicated cases it may be better to operate, directly realign the pieces, and hold them together with plates and screws.

Once everything is in position, your body can start to repair itself. It does this by forming little bridges of bone across the fracture. The new bone is fragile. If you disrupt it by putting too much pressure on the healing site, the new bone will break, and you'll be back to square one. The more you disrupt the new bone, the slower it grows, and if you continually interrupt the healing process, it will eventually come to a complete stop. You can see why it is so important to follow your doctor's advice about activity and try not to do more than they recommend.

Unlike acute fractures, stress fractures tend to come on gradually. The repetitive stress of high impact activities will cause microscopic breaks in your bones. Under normal circumstances, you'll repair these small cracks while you rest, but if you're pounding the pavement every day, the cracks won't get a chance to heal and they will get bigger. You'll start to develop pain, and if the pounding continues, your stress fracture will progress to the point where the bone has a complete break. The risk factors for stress fractures include:

> High impact activities
> Stress/recovery imbalance
> Weak bones, poor nutrition, and/or loss of menstrual periods
> Poor shock-absorbing equipment
> Hard surfaces

Stress fractures occur most commonly in the lower extremities but can also occur in the upper extremities and the spine (Knapp 1997). Early stress fractures may be difficult to diagnose because the X-ray abnormalities may take a couple of weeks to develop. Your doctor will need to advise you of the best course of action if a stress fracture is suspected.

Ligament Injuries

Ligaments hold your bones together at your joints. They work like ropes that extend from one bone to the next to stabilize your joints and allow them to move in very specific ways. Take your knee for example. It works like a hinge that can move back and forth in one basic direction. When you are standing with your legs straight, your lower leg can swing backward but it can't move from side to side. If you wanted to move your leg from side to side, you would have to move your entire leg from the hip.

The reason that you can't move your lower leg to the side when your leg is straight is that there are two ligaments on either side of your knee that keep the bones from moving in that direction. They are called the medial and lateral collateral ligaments. The knee also contains two other important ligaments known as the anterior and posterior cruciate ligaments. They are found inside the knee, and they keep the two main bones that meet at the knee from moving backward and forward in relation to each other.

You'll take your ligaments for granted until someone comes slamming into you and forces your knee to move in the wrong direction. You can get three types of ligament injuries. If the ligament is strained but there is no appreciable change in its length, it is called a Grade I strain. Once you let it heal, it should work like the original equipment as long as there were no other significant injuries.

In a Grade II strain, the fibers of the ligament are stretched and partially torn. This type of injury will also heal with proper treatment, but your knee will move in ways that it doesn't like to because the ligament can be a little longer than usual. The resulting instability can eventually damage other structures in your knee because as the bones move into awkward positions, they'll put more pressure on the cartilage in your knee. Since some of the ligament fibers are torn, the remaining ligament may be weaker and susceptible to further injury.

A Grade III ligament injury occurs when the force is so great that it completely ruptures the fibers of the ligament. A common example of a ruptured ligament is a ruptured anterior cruciate ligament of the knee. It will not heal by itself no matter how hard you try. With an injury like this you'll probably be able to do many of your basic activities like walking or even running in a straight line, but without an intact anterior cruciate ligament your knee will feel unstable when you plant your foot to change directions. The two bones of the knee will slide back and forth on each other giving you an eerie, painful feeling as they stress the other structures in your knee. This type of repetitive stress can result in serious long-term problems with your knee, and most young athletes who sustain this type of injury will choose to surgically reconstruct the ligament.

Your ankle is another area that is at risk for ligament injuries. When you twist your ankle, you can disrupt the ligaments that hold it together. Many athletes will twist their ankle and then hobble around for days or even weeks before getting it looked at. By then it is usually quite swollen, and they have gotten off on the wrong foot for a complete and rapid recovery. You can improve your recovery time by getting an early exam to confirm that you don't have a serious injury. With the correct diagnosis, you can get started on the right treatment. The typical approach to an ankle sprain involves early treatment with compression and immobilization followed by specific rehabilitation exercises. It seems like overkill at first, but if you don't give your ligaments their best chance for a full recovery, you can be looking at a weak ankle for a lifetime.

You can decrease your chances of an ankle injury by improving your strength and proprioception (your sense of position). Writing the alphabet with your toes or balancing on a bonga board—a board that sits on top of a ball or rolling pin—can help you develop a better sense of how your foot and ankle are positioned. That way if it starts to move the wrong way, you will quickly sense it, adjust your position, and hopefully avoid an injury. Taping your ankle also helps you to sense when it is moving the wrong way so that you can make the adjustments that will keep you from getting hurt. Both taping and proprioceptive exercises are an important part of rehabilitating an injured ankle and preventing further injury.

Muscle and Tendon Injuries

Muscle and tendon injuries are some of the most common injuries that athletes experience. They typically occur when the muscle is suddenly stretched or loaded beyond its capacity. The result is microscopic tearing along the muscle fiber, particularly at the muscle-tendon junction.

Although a sudden overload is a frequent cause of muscle tears, you can also get microscopic tears in your muscles when you have a hard workout. Exercises that involve eccentric muscle contractions are notorious for causing muscle breakdown and a delayed onset of muscle soreness. As you recall, eccentric muscle contractions are when the muscle actually gets longer while it's being loaded. Running downhill or landing from a jump are good examples of activities that require eccentric muscle contractions.

When you injure your muscles, your immune system needs to step in to begin the repair process. As your immune system triggers the inflammatory response, you'll start to experience pain, swelling, and tenderness. The greater the damage, the more inflammation you'll experience and the longer it will take to heal. The bottom line is that sore muscles and tendons are weaker and susceptible to severe injury from seemingly trivial workloads (Garrett 1996).

If you get enough rest, you'll rebuild your muscles and tendons in a way that makes them stronger. The usual treatment involves rest, ice, and gentle massage. Actively moving the muscle through its range of motion will also help with the recovery process (Best 1997). There is no specific formula for how long to rest because every injury is different. *You just need to listen to your body and let the amount of pain you are having guide you.* We'll talk more about muscle and tendon injuries when we talk about chronic injuries.

Researchers have tried to identify factors that lead to acute injuries. They include fatigue, weakness, improper body mechanics, faulty equipment, dangerous conditions, stiffness, and difficulty with coordination. You can combat the effects of stiffness and difficulty with coordination by doing exercises that improve your flexibility and agility.

Agility can be defined as your ability to successfully respond to the immediate changes in your environment and body position. This requires dynamic stabilization of your joints by rapid, coordinated muscle contractions. You can improve your agility by performing agility drills (Wojtys 1996). These include:

1. Slideboarding drills
2. Unilateral bounding box hop jumps
3. Foot crossover drills
4. Figure of eight running drills
5. Backward running

Flexibility also plays a role in injury prevention. In sports like gymnastics and martial arts, you have to be flexible just to participate. We just saw how you can injure your muscles when they are suddenly stretched beyond their capacity. You can see why flexible muscles will tolerate more stretch before they are injured (Garrett 1996). Flexible athletes also respond better to activities requiring eccentric muscle contractions (McHugh 1999).

Since stretching improves flexibility, you'll want to make it part of your routine. Many athletes stretch at the beginning of their workout as part of their warm-up. You can do it whenever it suits you, but a comfortable stretch can be a soothing part of your recovery from a hard workout. A good stretch and massage at the end of your workout can also prevent soreness by mobilizing the lactic acid in your muscles.

The way you stretch is important because if you stretch your muscles too hard, it can actually increase your risk for injury (Garrett 1996). Try to maintain a comfortable, slow, steady stretch for a count of five to ten seconds. Avoid bouncing and other quick movements while you stretch and don't forget to breathe.

Head Injuries

I want to mention a few words about head injuries because they are relatively common, and the results can be devastating. Any head injury resulting in loss of consciousness or a change in level of consciousness requires prompt medical evaluation. This includes the common episode where the athlete "gets their bell rung" or is temporarily dazed by a hard blow to the head. When these injuries occur on the field, you need to be careful not to move the athlete because a hard blow to the head can also cause serious neck injuries. Experienced medical or paramedical personnel should evaluate the athlete on the field because if you move someone with a spinal cord injury without properly supporting their neck, you can do further, irreversible damage.

If the mechanism of injury or the symptoms suggest a significant head or neck injury, the athlete should be moved with a backboard only after the head and neck have been properly stabilized and only by experienced personnel. If the athlete is wearing a helmet, it's better to leave it on until they receive medical attention.

You can never be faulted for calling the paramedics for assistance if you suspect the possibility of a significant head or neck injury. In this case it is always better to err on the side of caution because head injuries can be confusing at times. The athlete may get a strong blow to the head and become dazed or even unconscious. When they awaken, they might seem to be fine and may want to continue playing. Don't allow this to happen. Some head injuries can result in delayed swelling or internal bleeding. The athlete may have a lucid interval where they seem to be fine only to rapidly deteriorate within minutes, hours, or days.

An athlete that receives a strong blow to the head needs to be evaluated by a physician to see if there are any signs of impending danger. Even if the athlete appears fine in the exam room, the physician will inform them and their family members of the sign and symptoms that warrant further evaluation. These include vomiting, headache, drowsiness, changes in behavior, changes in vision, blurred vision, double vision, unequal pupils, and numbness or weakness.

If the patient falls asleep, they need to be awakened several times during the first night to make sure that they haven't deteriorated.

Second Impact Syndrome is another serious complication of a head injury and it can occur days or even weeks after the symptoms of the first head injury have resolved. The scenario typically begins with a strong blow to the head that results in loss of consciousness or dazing. The athlete starts to recover or only may have mild residual symptoms such as headache or nausea. As they are starting to feel better, they resume their activity, and a second, relatively mild head impact leads to unexpected, devastating consequences. Unfortunately, the initial impact causes brain swelling and instability of the blood vessels that supply the brain. Since the brain is enclosed in a rigid skull, there is no room for further swelling from another impact. The result can be brain damage and death. This syndrome occurs most commonly in boxing and football, but it can occur in any sport where you can get hit in the head, including if you are just horsing around.

In general, any athlete that has had a significant head injury needs to be protected from subsequent injury for a minimum of two weeks even if they have no residual symptoms. If he has residual symptoms like nausea, numbness, or headache, he may need to wait longer depending on the severity of his injury (Cantu 1998). All head injuries with altered mental status or residual symptoms need to be evaluated by a physician.

The best approach to managing head and neck injuries is to prevent them. One adage that certainly applies is to look before you leap. Many head and neck injuries occur when people dive into water that is too shallow. Occasionally the water is deep enough, but there may be a dangerous obstacle like a rock or pylon under the surface. In this situation looking from above is not enough, you have to actually get in the water and physically check out the entire area. One of my best friends ran into the water and noticed that it was getting deeper. He dove into a wave, hit his head on a shallow sand bar, and became a permanent quadriplegic. He wants me to remind you to please look *and* thoroughly check out before you leap. It sounds like good advice.

Another valuable bit of advice is to watch where you are going. Many head and neck injuries occur when people run into another object. The object may be moving or stationary. Trees, goal posts, concrete walls, cars, and even other people are all very hard when you run into them. It is a good idea to take a moment and survey your sports area from the perspective of safety because safety is everyone's responsibility. If you've identified a potentially dangerous situation, take it upon yourself to see that it is corrected or at least clearly marked and padded. Regardless, you will want to watch where you are going because objects move and even padded walls and goalposts can be dangerous when you run into them at full speed. I know this all seems like common sense, but you would be surprised at how often these types of injuries occur.

Helmets are becoming a standard in any sport that places the athlete at risk for head injury. A properly designed helmet can absorb much of the shock from an impact and provide a substantial reduction of head injury. Please note that I said substantial reduction. A helmet is not foolproof and should not give you the false sense of security that allows you to be careless. One example is an athlete that leads with their head because they are wearing a helmet. This practice is called spearing, and it is prohibited in football and other contact sports. Even with a helmet, the force transmitted through the helmet can injure your head and neck. The combination of good technique, proper equipment (helmets and neck supports), and appropriate cervical strengthening exercises can help prevent both permanent and temporary head and neck injuries (Cross 2003).

Good equipment can help to protect you from injury, but defective equipment can cause substantial injuries. A frayed brake cable on your bike or a faulty ski binding can result in a lot of pain and suffering. When it comes to safety-related equipment, don't cut corners. Be sure to regularly inspect your equipment for signs of wear and replace worn parts before they break. Remember, your life could depend on it.

Eye Injuries

Corneal abrasions are scratches in the outer layers of the eye. Relatively small objects like a finger or even a speck of sand can scratch the cornea. When this happens, you'll know that something has gone wrong because it is very uncomfortable.

You'll want to go to your doctor to confirm the diagnosis, and early treatment can make a big difference in the length of recovery. The good news is that these injuries will usually heal within twenty-four hours if properly treated. The best approach is always prevention, and in this case it means wearing the appropriate eye protection for your sport.

Retinal detachments result from a blow to the eye from a midsize object like a finger, elbow, or racquetball. Racquetball and squash are particularly high risk because of the size of the ball and the speed at which it travels. There is usually some degree of visual impairment although it may not be immediately apparent. Early evaluation and treatment can prevent permanent visual disturbance and blindness. Wearing the correct type of eye protection is a must in any sport that puts you at risk for a blow to the eye from a medium-sized object.

Blowout fractures result from a blow to the rim of the eye from an object that is larger than the rim. A fist, baseball, or knee can cause this type of injury. The result is a fracture of the orbit of the eye and can lead to visual changes as well as disruption of the full range of eye motion. Eyewear can provide some degree of protection, but the best type of protection is usually attached to a helmet in the form of a facemask or shield.

Ultraviolet light can cause both temporary or permanent visual disturbance and blindness. Snow, water, and other highly reflective surfaces can substantially increase your level of exposure to ultraviolet (UV) radiation. Glasses that provide high levels of UV protection are mandatory for sports like skiing, snowboarding, mountain climbing, and sailing. In addition, UV protection may protect you from developing cataracts and cancers of the eye.

Abdominal Injuries

The abdomen is another area where it can be difficult to assess the level of injury so I just want to make you aware of some of the potential problems. Hopefully this will help you make the right decision when you or one of your friends gets hit in the abdomen.

The main problem with abdominal injuries is internal bleeding. Your liver and spleen can be lacerated, but you won't be able to see that you are losing blood because it is collecting inside your abdominal cavity. If the bleeding continues, you'll become weak and eventually you'll pass out. Unfortunately, by this point you have lost a substantial amount of blood, and by the time someone gets you to the hospital you can be in shock.

With a substantial blow to the abdomen, it is better to get checked out right away. This is true even if the person gets up and tells you that they are okay. It can take quite a while to get to the hospital, get through the triage desk, obtain a diagnosis, assemble a surgical team, and get to the organ to stop the bleeding. Every year athletes die from blunt abdominal injuries and unrecognized internal bleeding. You don't want to be one of them.

Mononucleosis is a condition that can predispose you to internal bleeding. It is a viral infection that mimics tonsillitis, but in half the cases the spleen becomes enlarged and can stay that way for up to five months. Even with a minor abdominal injury, a large spleen can be susceptible to rupture and bleeding. Athletes with a recent history of mononucleosis should not participate in sports for at least four weeks (*Handbook of Adolescent Medicine* 2003) and they should not participate in contact sports (including just horsing around) until a doctor determines that their spleen is not enlarged (Peter 1998).

Preventing splenic rupture in athletes with mono is straightforward as long as the correct diagnosis is made. In many cases, the correct diagnosis is not established because the tonsillitis may not be severe or it's attributed to another cause. It's a good idea to get checked out by a doctor if you are feeling unusually tired or have a sore throat that doesn't go away in a couple of days.

Chronic Injuries

As you might imagine, chronic injuries tend to persist. They can come on gradually from overuse, or they can start as an acute injury that has never had the opportunity to fully heal. Regardless of how the injury starts, the usual culprit is repetitive trauma. Some part of your body gets irritated and before the repair job is complete you go out and damage it again. The two main factors that lead to chronic injury are excess stress and inadequate recovery (sound familiar?).

Taking on more than you can handle can perpetuate a chronic injury, but overtraining isn't always the culprit. Poor body mechanics can increase the forces on specific body parts causing injuries with relatively light workloads. If you are having problems with a chronic injury, you may want to systematically review each of the following areas with your doctor and trainer to be sure that you are doing everything possible to correct the problem. The main factors contributing to poor body mechanics include:

- Structural abnormalities that can be genetic, age related, or caused by previous injuries
- Muscle strength imbalances
- Poor technique
- Faulty or incorrectly suited equipment

Structural abnormalities

We are all built a little differently, and some of us are more suited for certain activities than others. You may have excessive pronation (a rotation of certain foot bones inward and downward), increasing the stress on your lower leg when you run, while your friend may have wide hips and knocked knees, placing increased stress on her kneecaps. Regardless of the problem, if you repetitively overstress a specific body part, it will result in a chronic injury.

In some cases you can make adjustments in your equipment to compensate for a structural abnormality. A custom-designed, rigid insert called an orthotic can decrease unnecessary motion in you foot and leg. This can dramatically decrease the amount of stress on your knee and lower leg. Occasionally exercises that strengthen specific muscle groups can help control excessive pressure on a body part. Your sports medicine doctor can work with you to get around some of these types of problems.

Age-Related Structural Weaknesses

Children and adolescents have skeletons that are not fully matured and the growth plates are not as strong as solid, calcified bone. Additionally, many major tendons are attached to areas of developing bone. In the face of repetitive stress, the bone and tendon become inflamed and actually begin to separate from the rest of the bone at the area of growth. This type of problem occurs most commonly in three areas of the body:

1.   Elbow: Little League Elbow, where the inner part of the elbow is repetitively stressed.
2.   Knee: Osgood-Shlater Disease occurs in sports that involve running and jumping. The patellar tendon can begin to separate from its attachment on the tibia.
3.   Foot: Sever's Disease also occurs in running and jumping sports but affects the heel bone.

If you suspect any of these problems, you'll want to see a sports physician before you develop a permanent problem. The treatment typically involves limiting the offending activity and increasing recovery time.

Injury-Related Structural Weaknesses

Ligament damage causes joint instability, and when your bones move in ways they are not supposed to, it will place excess pressure on the joint surface and its surrounding structures. If the problem goes uncorrected, you can cause permanent damage. These types of problems are common in people with severe ankle sprains and ruptured anterior cruciate ligaments. If you are not a candidate for reconstruction, then bracing and strengthening exercises may provide some stability.

Muscle Imbalances

Many of the muscles in your body work in opposing directions. Your biceps flex your arm and your triceps extend your arm. Some activities will favor the development of one of the opposing muscle groups leading to an imbalance in the strength between the opposing sides. Exercises that can strengthen the weaker side can help you maintain balanced strength and prevent possible injuries.

Equipment

Faulty or poorly suited equipment can also contribute to repetitive trauma. A bike seat that is too low can place increased stress on your kneecap. Worn-out running shoes cause excessive foot motion and increase the stress on your lower leg and knee. Ski bindings that don't release at the right time can also place a great deal of pressure on your lower extremities.

Be sure that your equipment is best suited for your size and ability. If you are developing a chronic injury, it is important to perform a thorough assessment of your equipment to see if you can make adjustments that will relieve some stress on the injured part of your body.

Technique

Sometimes the way that you perform a particular activity can put excess stress on your body. Not having the right timing, position, and leverage can greatly increase the forces on isolated parts of your body. We see this with tennis players that "wrist" their backhands and injure their elbows. Having an experienced instructor evaluate your technique can help you make corrections that decrease the stress on your body.

Overuse injuries

The main cause of chronic injury is overuse. Repetitive microtrauma can cause specific injury patterns called overuse injuries. Many of these problems begin as minor inflammation, but if you don't take the proper corrective action, they can progress to serious long-term problems (Barry 1996). In the early stages, most of these injuries can be treated with conservative measures including rest, ice, and correction of biomechanical and training problems.

I've put together a short list of the more common overuse injuries so that you can have an idea of the problems you might run into. Keep in mind that this is a basic review to help you identify a developing injury during the early stages so you can get the help of your sports physician before you develop a permanent problem. Do not try to manage and treat your injuries without the help of a professional.

Epicondylitis: One of the reasons that your hands work so well is that most of the muscles that control your hands and fingers are in your arms. These muscles have long tendons that cross the wrist and attach at various points along your hands and fingers. Some of the muscles that control your hand also cross the elbow and attach on the prominent ends of the upper bone of the arm called the epicondyles. These muscles play an important role in gripping and stabilizing your hand and wrist. They are important in sports that require gripping, throwing, or hitting with a racquet or club.

One of the most common overuse injuries at the elbow is lateral epicondylitis or "tennis elbow." In addition to racquet sports, this problem can occur in any sport that requires gripping, such as weightlifting, martial arts, and gymnastics. Sometimes even seemingly light activities like typing, playing the piano, or using your mouse can aggravate this problem and get in the way of your recovery.

During the early stages, you'll experience pain and inflammation in the outer side of your elbow during activity. If you continue with the offending activity, you might notice that it will start to hurt when you grip anything. Even a handshake can become a painful experience for people with this problem.

In uncomplicated cases, rest, ice, and massage can alleviate the symptoms. If you are a tennis player, the solution may be as simple as changing the size of the grip on your racquet, easing the tension on your strings, or reevaluating your technical approach. If your symptoms persist, you'll want to see a doctor who specializes in sports medicine so that they can confirm the diagnosis and recommend the appropriate treatment. Typically this will involve stretching and strengthening exercises, a tennis elbow support, and anti-inflammatory medicine. In resistant cases a cortisone injection can provide long-term relief with relatively little risk of side effects.

You'll want to take care of this problem in the early stages because with chronic irritation you can develop permanent changes in the surface of the bone that can only be treated surgically.

Throwing sports and forehand swings in racquet sports can also irritate the medial aspect of your elbow causing *medial epicondylitis*. This is also called golfer's elbow because a poorly executed golf swing can place a high amount of stress on your medial elbow. The basic approach to treatment is similar to tennis elbow. You'll want to get this problem under control in the early stages because the nerve running along the inside of your elbow travels close to the medial epicondyle, and chronic inflammation in this area can lead to nerve irritation (Barry 1996).

Impingement syndrome: Every time you bring your arm up over your head a group of muscles at the top of your arm need to slide under the bones that form the upper part of your shoulder. This group of muscles is called the rotator cuff, and they play an important role in stabilizing your arm at the shoulder.

The supraspinatus muscle forms the upper aspect of the rotator cuff. It's a tight squeeze for the supraspinatus, and repeated overhead activities in throwing sports, basketball, volleyball, and swimming can lead to inflammation of the muscle tendon and it's protective bursa. To complicate matters, in some people the bones that are above the supraspinatus hook downward, making it harder for it to glide back and forth.

For mild symptoms you can resort to rest and ice, but if your symptoms persist, you'll be better-off getting the help of your physician because continued aggravation of the tendon can wear it down to the point where it tears. Once you tear the rotator cuff, you'll have to choose between surgery and a permanently weak shoulder.

The typical medical treatment for impingement syndrome involves rest, ice, and anti-inflammatory medicines. In resistant cases, a cortisone injection can be very effective in relieving inflammation.

Stretching and strengthening also play an important role in the prevention and rehabilitation of this problem. You can strengthen your rotator cuff by doing internal and external rotation exercises with an elastic band. Your trainer or physical therapist can show you exactly how to do these exercises. Not only do these exercises help with prevention and rehabilitation, but they have also been shown to improve performance in some overhead sports (Trieber et al. 1998).

Patello-femoral syndrome: Your quads are hard at work every time you squat, jump, or land. They are the strongest muscle group in your body, and the force from your quadriceps gets transferred across your knee to your lower leg via the patella (kneecap) and patellar tendon. Your kneecap has two sides, the side that you feel under your skin, and the opposite side that presses up against your femur. It's this side that has to glide back and forth along the groove at the end of your femur whenever you bend your knee. If it doesn't track properly, you'll get pain and inflammation on the backside of your kneecap.

Rest and ice can alleviate some of the symptoms, but if they persist, you'll want to have an expert look at your biomechanics so that you can correct the underlying problem. Your doctor may also want to send you to a physical therapist for some strengthening exercises that are specifically designed to correct some of the muscle imbalances that are common with patello-femoral syndrome. Finally, you can alleviate some of the strain on your kneecap by minimizing the amount of pronation in your foot with an orthotic.

It's important to get this problem treated in the early stages because if you continue to grind down your patella, you'll damage the cartilage that gives the patella its nice, smooth surface. This is called chondromalacia. It's a relatively permanent condition, and it's difficult to treat even with surgery.

Shin splints: Many athletes use the term shin splints to describe pain in the front part of their lower leg. Actually there are several distinct syndromes that can cause pain in this part of your body. The most common are Medial Tibial Stress Syndrome, Anterior Compartment Syndrome, and stress fractures (Wilder 2004). We've already talked about stress fractures earlier in this chapter, so I'm just going to focus on the other two.

Medial Tibial Stress Syndrome is an irritation along the medial side of your tibia. This is where some of the muscles that control the motion of your foot attach to the bone. The irritation is usually caused by running and is more common in people with excessive pronation.

Rest and ice can help, but the best solution is to correct the underlying problem. Since pronation is the main offender, one of the best ways to treat this problem is to wear a good supportive shoe or to get an orthotic insert that stabilizes your foot.

It can be difficult to tell the difference between Medial Tibial Stress Syndrome and a stress fracture, so you'll want to see your doctor if your symptoms last longer than a couple of days or if you have recurring symptoms.

The symptoms of an *Anterior Compartment Syndrome* begin with a dull ache along the lateral side of your tibia. In severe cases you can get numbness along your instep and a weak foot. The muscles in this part of your body are enclosed in a tough fibrous sheath with little room for swelling. If they become swollen from rapid growth, inflammation, or trauma, the pressure can be so great that it cuts off the circulation to the muscle.

Continued swelling can compress the nerve that runs through the muscle. That's what causes the numbness and weakness. This is not the kind of problem that you want to be dealing with on your own, so if you are having pain in this part of your body, you'll want to get it checked out right away.

Achilles tendonitis: The Achilles tendon is the strongest tendon in your body. It connects your calf muscles to your heel bone and plays a critical role in running, jumping, and landing. With repetitive stress, the tendon becomes inflamed, and you'll have pain and tenderness in the area just above the point where your tendon attaches to your heel bone. Unfortunately, the lack of blood supply to this area tends to make the healing process slower. Rest and ice can help in the early stages, but if your symptoms persist, you'll want to see your doctor right away because chronic Achilles tendonitis is hard to treat and an irritated, weakened tendon is more likely to rupture.

Typically the treatment involves relative rest, heel lifts, and changing your training program to minimize running, jumping, and landing. Your doctor may also recommend an oral anti-inflammatory medication, but they will avoid using cortisone injections because they can weaken the tendon.

Plantar Fasciitis: Your plantar fascia is a tough, fibrous tissue that runs along the bottom of your foot from your heel bone to your forefoot. It helps you stabilize your foot when you push off from your heel to the ball of your foot.

You'll know that you've irritated your plantar fascia when you get up in the morning and feel like you've bruised your heel. The pain frequently improves with activity but comes back after you've been off your feet for a while. Your first inclination might be to pad your heel, and although this might give you some relief, it doesn't fully address the underlying problem.

The inflammation in your heel isn't from compression of your heel as much as it is from your plantar fascia tugging at your heel bone. The treatment typically involves rest, taping, and supportive shoes. If your symptoms don't improve with basic care, your doctor may also recommend an anti-inflammatory medication, an orthotic insert, or a cortisone injection.

Overtraining

One of the main culprits in each of these chronic injuries is overtraining. You already know that this means too much work and not enough rest. I want to mention it again because it is closely related to some of the closing comments that I want to make. The issue of how hard you train gets us back to some of the points that we talked about at the beginning of this book. They include having an understanding of what's motivating you.

Today's athletes are being pushed to train harder than ever. Gymnastics, soccer, dance, and martial arts seem to go on indefinitely from year to year. Summer leagues, clubs, and special training camps now connect seasonal sports so that they become year-round activities. In some areas these types of programs are an unwritten requirement for getting on a school team. The result is that kids are training and competing under pressure for most of the year. They will play through an ankle injury during the off-season because they don't want to disappoint anyone. The result: a loose ankle that is chronically swollen and painful. When the important season comes around, they are not at 100%, and the slightest twist puts them on the bench for a month.

Some of my young patients are relieved when I tell them that they need to take some time off. It may be the only graceful way for them to take a much-needed break. Other athletes are afraid to seek medical attention because of retaliation from their coach for being sick or injured. I've even seen coaches go as far as overriding a physician's recommendations and insist that a sick or injured athlete show up for practice.

I can go on with examples, but what it boils down to is the belief that pushing harder is always better and that sport participation is all work and no play. Some coaches and parents seem to believe that everyone is on a track to the big time and that we need to risk everything to get there. To the contrary, if we have an athlete with true potential, we need to encourage internal motivation and then focus on pacing and protecting them from burnout and injury.

For the rest of us, participation in sports is about staying in shape and having fun. Okay, bragging rights are also important. Perhaps with a more relaxed attitude toward early sports development, we'll learn to associate athletic activity with fitness and pleasure instead of pain and pressure. The end result will be better top-level athletes and fewer couch potatoes.

I hope what you've learned from reading this book will give you a better perspective so that you can train smarter, know when to push harder, and know when it's time for a break.

APPENDIX A

Key Terms

Achilles tendonitis. Inflammation in the tendon that connects the calf muscle to the heel bone.

acute mountain sickness. Illness caused by a person's difficulty in acclimating to high altitude.

aerobic. Activity or metabolism in the presence of oxygen.

amino acids. Building blocks that make up proteins.

anemia. A condition characterized by a low red blood cell concentration that is frequently, but not always, caused by iron deficiency.

anaerobic. Activity or metabolism in the absence of oxygen.

anaerobic threshold. The transition from aerobic metabolism to anaerobic metabolism where the body outpaces its ability to deliver oxygen, and starts to produce higher levels of lactic acid.

anterior compartment syndrome. Swelling that produces a dull ache along the lateral side of the tibia.

ATP (adenosine triphosphate). A molecule that is the main energy source for muscle contraction during prolonged exercise.

blowout fracture. A fracture of the eye's orbit resulting from a blow to the rim of the eye by an object that is larger than the rim. It can lead to visual changes and affect the full range of eye motion.

branched-chain amino acids. A subset of essential amino acids needed for the maintenance of muscle tissue. They include leucine, isoleucine, and valine and in supplement form, they are sometimes marketed as performance-enhancing agents.

carbohydrates. Molecules that are the primary fuel source for athletic activity. They include sugars, starches, and fiber.

chondromalacia. Cartilage damage caused by continual grinding down of the patella.

concentric muscle contraction. Movement causing the muscle length to shorten during activity.

conduction. An exchange or transfer of heat through motion.

corneal abrasions. Scratches in the outer layers of the eye.

cross-training. Training program that utilizes multiple activities to improve endurance and cardiovascular fitness without the repetitive trauma.

eccentric muscle contraction. Movement that lengthens a muscle during an activity.

endurance. The ability to sustain a given task without fatiguing.

enzymes. Specialized proteins that control thousands of essential chemical reactions in the body.

epicondylitis. Inflammation in the either side of the elbow; sometimes called "tennis elbow" on the lateral elbow or "golfer's elbow" on the medial side of the elbow.

evaporation. A process by which water on the skin becomes airborne water vapor.

external visual imagery. To imagine oneself performing the task as though you were an observer.

Female Athletic Triad. A syndrome that includes disordered eating, loss of menstrual period, and thinning of the bones caused by an imbalance between stress and recovery.

free fatty acids. Chains of carbon and hydrogen with an organic acid group at one end of the molecule. They are one of the basic components of triglycerides.

free-form amino acids. Protein supplements that contain concentrated amounts of one or more specific amino acid. As with branched-chain amino acids, these compounds are sometimes marketed as performance-enhancing aids.

glycemic index. Guide used to help a person estimate how much insulin he or she will produce when eating a variety of carbohydrates.

gluconeogenesis. A backup response by the human body to glycogen depletion by scavenging protein molecules and converting them into a small amount of glucose.

glycogen. Long chains of glucose stored in the liver that can be used to maintain normal blood sugar levels during exercise.

glycolysis. A chemical process that breaks down glucose.

high altitude cerebral edema. A swelling of brain tissue that can occur in accelerated cases of acute mountain sickness and high altitude pulmonary edema.

high altitude pulmonary edema. An accumulation of fluid in the lung tissue caused by rapidly ascending to altitudes above 8,000 feet.

hydrogenation. A process that manipulates the saturation of a fatty acid by adding hydrogen to the carbon double bonds of a polyunsaturated fat.

hydrolysates. Proteins that have been broken down into smaller chains of one, two, or three amino acids.

hyperventilation Breathing more rapidly than necessary. It should be avoided before activity, especially before lifting and then holding one's breath in a weight-lifting workout.

hypothermia. An abnormally low body temperature that requires medical attention.

impingement syndrome. The pinching a group of muscles that makes up the rotator cuff in the shoulder.

insulin. A hormone that regulates blood sugar in the body.

intensity. The amount of power (force multiplied by velocity) used to perform the given task. High force multiplied by high velocity = high intensity.

internal visual imagery. To visualize the performance from the perspective of the performer.

isokinetic. Implies that the speed at which the weight is being moved will remain constant.

isometric. Implies that there is no change in the length of the muscle as force and resistance are applied.

isotonic. Implies that the level of resistance is maintained at a constant level.

kinesthetic imagery. The athlete is trying to feel what it's like to perform complex motor tasks, such as in diving and gymnastics.

lactic acid. A compound made during glycolysis in anaerobic conditions. Accumulation of lactic acid is one of the factors leading to muscle fatigue.

leverage. Proper body position in relation to an adjacent object or opponent that gives an athlete an advantage in competition.

maximal oxygen consumption (VO2max). The point at which a person has reached the maximal exercise capacity that can be measured in terms of the maximal amount of oxygen that person can use.

medial epicondylitis. Inflammation of the medial aspect of the elbow; often called "golfer's elbow."

medial tibial stress syndrome. Irritation along the medial side of the tibia, where some of the muscles that control the motion of the foot attach to the bone.

minerals. Basic elements that exist as ionic salts.

momentum. The tendency during an athletic activity to stay in a particular motion.

mononucleosis. A viral infection that causes swollen tonsils, fatigue, and can enlarge the spleen for up to five months.

monounsaturated fats. Fats that contain a double bond in their carbon chain and can lower LDL cholesterol.

osteoporosis. A common thinning and weakening of the bones that occurs in women as they age.

oxygen debt. The abrupt decrease in oxygen level at the start of exercise.

parameterization. The process of learning to apply a skill in a variety of settings.

patello-femoral syndrome. Pain and inflammation on the backside of your knee-cap, caused by the kneecap not tracking properly.

percent of repetition maximum (%RM). The percentage of one's 1-RM that is being lifted. For example, if one's 1-RM for the bench press is 200 pounds, a workout with ten repetitions at 50%RM would be set to 100 pounds.

periodization. A training cycle that prepares the athlete for intense competition by breaking the year down into various stages of training.

placebo effect. An effect in which patients administered a pill not containing actual medicine begin to feel different because of the perception they are receiving the real medicine.

plantar fasciitis. Irritation of a tough, fibrous tissue that runs along the bottom of the foot from the heel bone to the forefoot.

plyometrics. Exercises that typically load and lengthen a muscle before the direction of contraction rapidly changes.

polypeptides: Intact proteins from milk, whey, egg, or soy.

polyunsaturated fats. Fats that have multiple carbon double bonds and are liquids at room temperature.

power. The product of force and velocity. It describes the ability to generate force as a factor of speed (force x velocity).

prehabilitation. A preventive exercise program that strengthens muscles, which are vulnerable to injury, before they are injured.

preloading. Stretching muscles to the appropriate length to take out slack before loading the muscle.

proprioceptive feedback. Sensory information that indicates where one's body parts are in relationship to each other.

prostaglandins. Chemicals that have hormonelike effects on blood vessels and intestines.

pyruvate. A molecule produced during the breakdown of glucose. In aerobic conditions, the body uses it to obtain ATP, whereas in anaerobic conditions it is converted to lactic acid.

radiation: An exchange of heat in the form of waves.

repetitions (reps). The number of times that an exercise or activity is being performed during a set.

repetition maximum (RM). The maximal amount of weight that a person can lift in a defined number of repetitions. 1-RM would be the maximal amount of weight that could be lifted during a specific activity one time. 5-RM would be the maximal amount of weight that could be lifted in five repetitions.

repetition maximum equivalent. An estimate of 1-RM based on the following formula: (Weight Lifted multiplied by Number of Repetitions multiplied 0.03) + Weight Lifted = 1-RM equivalent. (Landers 1985).

retinal detachment. An injury that causes the membrane lining the eye, the retina, to separate from the underlying blood vessels.

saturated fats. Fats with each carbon atom sharing one electron with the adjacent carbon and the remaining electrons shared with two hydrogen atoms. These fats increase a person's risk of heart disease.

second impact syndrome. A serious complication of a head injury that is characterized by a subsequent injury after the initial impact.

sets. Groups of repetitions.

sickle-cell anemia. A disabling genetic condition affecting in which the recipient has abnormally shaped red blood cells.

sickle cell trait. One half of the genetic expression of the sickle-cell anemia gene. It doesn't cause sickle-cell anemia, but makes the recipient vulnerable to illness if they exercise after rapidly ascending to high elevations.

specificity. Workouts geared to target certain muscle groups or level of exertion used in a particular competition.

strength. The maximal force that a muscle or group of muscles can generate at a specific velocity.

stress fracture. A microscopic break in a bone frequently caused from repetitive, high impact exercise.

synergy. The coordinated effort of several muscle groups working in unison.

taper. A training method that reduces the intensity of workouts as a competition approaches to allow the body to regain full strength.

timing. Muscles firing at the precise moment to carry out a particular athletic movement.

triglycerides. A group of three fatty acids joined by a glyceride molecule. It is one of the forms in which fats are stored and transferred in your blood.

vitamins. Complex organic molecules that are typically found in foods and serve as essential cofactors in metabolism.

volume. The total amount of exercise performed during a period of time. In weight lifting it is the amount of weight lifted over a period of time. In general, high volume refers to more repetitions and more sets.

APPENDIX B

Chemical Structures of Some Sugars, and Fats

Monosaccharides: Disaccharides:

Glucose   Maltose

Galactose   Lactose

Fructose   Sucrose

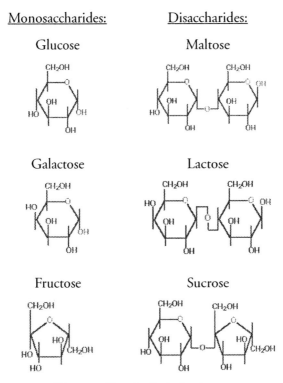

Figure 1 Simple Carbohydrates

Saturated fat:

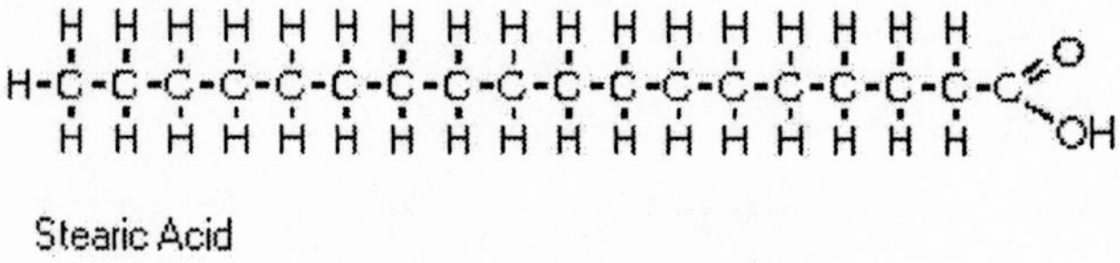

Stearic Acid

Monounsaturated fat:

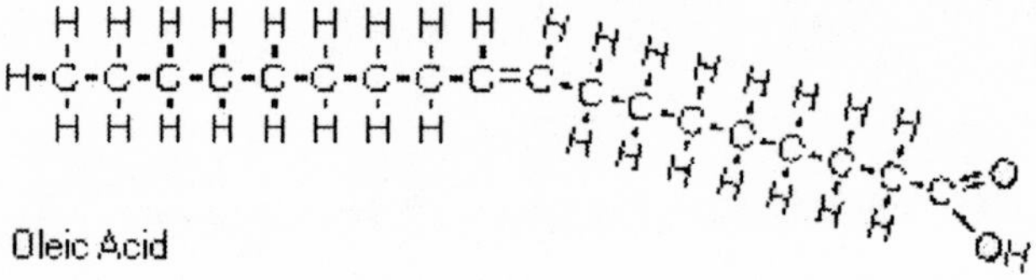

Oleic Acid

Polyunsaturated fat.:

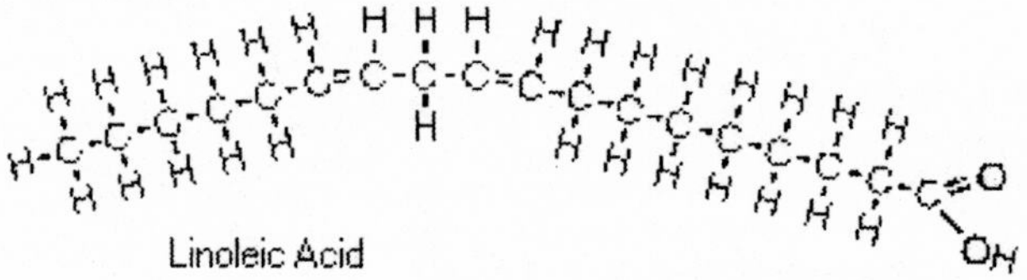

Linoleic Acid

Figure 2 Fats

Reference List

Sports Psychology

Adair, Robert. *The Physics of Baseball*. New York: HarperCollins Publishers, 1994.

Ahern, David. 1997. Psychosocial factors in sports injury rehabilitation. *Clinics in Sports Medicine* 16(4):755–768.

Cox, Richard H. *Sports Psychology*. Burr Ridge, IL: WCB/McGraw-Hill,1988.

Ellender, Lee. 2005. *Prim Care: Clinics in Office Practice* 32(1):277–92

Finkenberg, Mel. 1996. College students' perceptions of the purposes of sports. *Perceptual and Motor Skills* 82:19–22.

Greydanus, Donald. 2002. Sports doping in the adolescent athlete: The hope, hype, and hyperbole. *Pediatric Clinics of North America* 49(4):829–855.

Hackfort, Dieter.1996. The display of emotions in elite athletes. *American Journal of Sports Medicine* 24:6:PS0080–PS0084.

Halvari, Hallgeir. 1995. Trait and state anxiety before and after competitive performance. *Perceptual and Motor Skills* 81:1059–1074.

Hardy, Lew. 1992. Psychological stress, performance, and injury in sport. *British Medical Bulletin* 48:2:615–629.

Hardy, Lew. 1996. Knowledge and conscious control of motor actions under stress. *British Journal of Psychology* 87:621–636.

Iso-Aloha, S. E. 1995. Intrapersonal and interpersonal factors in athletic performance. *Scand J Med Sci Sports* 5:191–199.

Jackson, Susan. 1996. Toward a conceptual understanding of the flow experience in elite athletes. *Research Quarterly for Exercise and Sport* 67(1)76–90.

Loehr, James. *The New Toughness Training For Sports*. New York: Penguin, 1994.

Murphy, Michael, and Rhea A. White. *In The Zone*: *Transcendent Experiences in Sports* New York: Penguin/Arkana, 1995.

Roberts, G. C. 1996. Effects of goal orientation on achievement beliefs, cognition, and strategies in team sport. *Scand J Med Sci Sports* 6:46–56.

Sports Nutrition

Almond, Christopher et al. 2005. Hyponatremia among runners in the Boston Marathon, *NEJM* Volume 352:1550–1556.

ACSM. 1996. Position stand on fluid and electrolyte replacement. *Medicine and Science in Sports Exercise* 28(1):I–VII.

AFP. 2006. ACSM Recommendations for Endurance Athletes. *American Family Physician* 73(3):547.

Armstrong, Lawrence. 1996. Vitamin and mineral supplements as nutritional aids to exercise performance and health. *Nutritional Reviews* 54(4):S149–S158.

Bloch, Tama. 1999. Nutritional aspects of exercise: Dietary examples. *Clinics in Sports Medicine* 18(3):703–711.

Bohl, Caroline H. 2002. Magnesium and exercise. *Clinical Reviews in Food Science and Nutrition* 42(6):533–566.

Brandle, E. 1996. Effects of chronic dietary protein intake on the renal function of healthy subjects. *European Journal of Clinical Nutrition* 50:734–740.

Cheuvront, Samuel. 1999. The Zone Diet and athletic performance. *Sports Medicine* 27(4):213–228.

Clark, Nancy. *Nancy Clark's Sports Nutrition Guidebook.* Second edition. Champaign, Illinois: Human Kinetics, 1997.

Clarkson, Priscilla M. 1994. Trace mineral requirements for athletes. *International Journal of Sports Nutrition* 4:104–109.

Clarkson, Priscilla M. 1995. Exercise and mineral status of athletes: Calcium, magnesium, phosphorus, and iron. *Medicine and Science in Sports and Exercise* 27:831–843.

Fitts, Robert. 1996. Muscle fatigue: The cellular aspects. *American Journal of Sports Medicine* 24:6: PS00009–PS00013.

Grandjean, Ann. 1999. Nutritional requirements to increase lean body mass. *Clinics in Sports Medicine* 18(3):623–632.

Halbert, Steven. 1997. Diet and nutrition in primary care: From A to Z. *Primary Care: Clinics in Office Practice* 24(4):825–841.

Herbert, Victor, and Genell J. Subak-Sharpe (eds.). *Total Nutrition: The Only Guide You'll Ever Need.* New York: St. Martin's Press, 1995.

Hermila, H. 1996. Vitamin C and common cold incidence: A review of studies with subjects under heavy physical stress. *International Journal of Sports Medicine* 17:379–383.

Holroyd, Kenneth. 2003. Complementary and alternative treatments. *Neurology* 60(7):S58–S62.

Ivy, John L. July 1999. Role of carbohydrate in physical activity. *Clinics in Sports Medicine* 18(3) 469–484.

Jakeman, P. 1993. Effect of antioxidant vitamin supplementation on muscle function after eccentric exercise. *European Journal of Applied Physiology* 67(5):426–430.

Latzka, William. 1999. Nutritional aspects of exercise: Water and electrolyte requirements for exercise. *Clinics in Sports Medicine* 18(3):513–524.

Lemon, Peter. 1995. Do athletes need more dietary protein and amino acids? *International Journal of Sports Nutrition* 5:S31–S61.

Lemon, Peter. 1996. Is increased dietary protein necessary or beneficial for individuals with a physically active lifestyle? *Nutritional Reviews* 54(4):169–S175.

Liares, Maria Jose. 2004. Role of cellular magnesium in heath and disease. *Frontiers in Bioscience* (9):262–276.

Martin, Wade. 1997. Effects of endurance training on fatty acid metabolism during whole body exercise. *Medicine and Science in Sports and Exercise* 29(5):635–639.

Miller, Elizabeth. 1998. Adolescent medicine: Nutrition and diet-related problems. *Primary Care: Clinics in Office Practice* 25(1):193–210.

Nieman, David. 1999. Nutritional aspects of exercise: Nutrition, exercise, and immune system function. *Clinics in Sports Medicine* 18(3):537–545.

Rankin, Janet Walberg. 1999. Role of protein in exercise. *Clinics in Sports Medicine* 18(3):499–511.

Sherman, W. M. 1989. Effects of four-hour pre-exercise carbohydrate feedings on cycling performance. *Medicine and Science in Sports and Exercise* 21:598–604.

Stearns, D. M. 1995. A prediction of chromium (III) accumulation in humans from chromium dietary supplements. *FASEB J* 9(15):1650–1657.

Sears, Barry. *Enter The Zone.* Harper Collins, New York, NY, 1995.

Turcotte, Lorraine. July 1999. Role of fats in exercise. *Clinics in Sports Medicine* 18(3):485–498.

USDA. *Dietary Guidelines for Americans 2005.* Executive summary.

Williams, Melvin H. 1999. Facts and fallacies of purported ergogenic amino acid supplements. *Clinics in Sports Medicine* 18(3):633–649.

Aerobic Fitness

Antonutto, Guglielmo. 1995. The concept of lactate threshold. *The Journal of Sports Medicine and Physical Fitness* 35:6–12.

Boulay, Marcel R. 1997. Monitoring high intensity endurance exercise with heart rate and thresholds. *Medicine and Science in Sports and Exercise* 29(1):125–132.

Cahill, Bernard. 1997. The clinical importance of the anaerobic energy system and its assessment in human performance. *American Journal of Sports Medicine* 25(6):863–872.

Gaiga, Milena C. 1995. The effect of an aerobic interval training program on intermittent anaerobic performance. *Canadian Journal of Applied Physiology* 20(4):452–464.

Loat, Christopher. 1993. Relationship between lactate and ventilatory thresholds during prolonged exercise. *Sports Medicine* 15(2):104–115.

Myers, Jonathan. 1997. Dangerous curves: A perspective on exercise, lactate, and the anaerobic threshold. *Chest* 111:787–795.

O'Toole, M. 1995.Applied physiology of triathlon. *Sports Medicine* 19(4):251–267.

Shephard, Roy. *Exercise Physiology.* Philadelphia, PA: Decker Inc, 1987.

Stricker, Paul. 1998. Other ergogenic agents. *Clinics in Sports Medicine* 17(2):283–297.

Tanaka, Hirofumi. 1998. Impact of resistance training on endurance performance. *Sports Medicine* 25(3):191–200.

Strength Training

Baechle, Thomas R., and Rodger W. Earle (eds.). *Essentials of Strength and Conditioning.* Champaign, IL: Human Kinetics, 1994.

Barrett, Jean. 1990. Strength training for female athletes: A review of selected aspects. *Sports Medicine* 9(4):216–228.

Fleck, Stephen J. *Designing Resistance Training Programs.* Champaign, IL: Human Kinetics, 1997.

Hewett, T. E. 1996. Plyometric Training in Female Athletes. *American Journal of Sports Medicine* 24(6):765–773.

Holloway, J. B. 1990. Strength Training for Female Athletes. *Sports Medicine* 9(4):216–228.

Landers, J. 1985. Maximum based on reps. *National Strength and Conditioning Association Journal* 6:60–61.

Loud, Keith. October 2003. Primary care of the elite or elite-emulating adolescent athlete. *Adolescent Medicine* 14(3):647–661.

Moss, B. M. 1997. Effects of maximal effort strength training with different loads on dynamic strength, cross-sectional area, load-power, load-velocity relationships. *European Journal of Applied Physiology* 75:193–199.

Stone, M. H. 1991. Health and performance related potential of resistance training. *Sports Medicine* 11(4):210–231.

Webb, David R. 1990. Strength training in children and adolescents. *Pediatric Clinics of North America* 37(5):1187–1210.

Wilson, G. J. 1993. The optimal training load for the development of dynamic athletic performance. *Medicine and Science in Sports and Exercise* 25(11):1279–1286.

Environmental Conditions

ACSM, Armstrong, Lawrence. 1996. Heat and cold illness during distance running. *Medicine and Science in Sports and Exercise* 28(12):I–X.

ACSM Costill, David. 1996. Position stand on fluid and electrolyte replacement. *Medicine and Science in Sports and Exercise* 28(1):I–VII.

Binkley, Helen. 2002. National Athletic Trainers' Association position statement: Exertional heat illnesses. *J Athl Train* 37(3):329–343.

Bracker, Mark. 1992. Environmental and thermal injury. *Clinics in Sports Medicine* 11(2):419–436.

Broad, Elizabeth. 1996. Body weight changes and voluntary fluid intakes during training and competition sessions in team sports. *International Journal of Sports Nutrition* 6:306–320.

Doubt, Thomas. 1991. Physiology of exercise in the cold. *Sports Medicine* 11(6):367–381.

Fritz, Robert. 1989. Cold exposure injuries: Prevention and treatment. *Clinics In Sports Medicine* 8(1):111–127.

Guyton, Arthur. *Textbook of Medical Physiology.* Philadelphia: W. B. Saunders Company, 1996.

Lugo-Amador, Nannette. May 2004. Heat-related illness. *Emergency Medicine Clinics of North America* 22(2):315–327.

Maughan, R. J. 1993. Fluid replacement in sport and exercise—a consensus statement. *British Journal of Sports Medicine* 27:1.

Maughan, R. J. 1994. Fluid replacement requirements in soccer. *Journal of Sports Science* 12:S29–S34.

Morton, Paul. May 2004. Wilderness survival. *Emergency Medicine Clinics of North America* 22(2):539–559.

Murray, Robert. 1995. Fluid needs in hot and cold environments. *International Journal of Sports Nutrition* 5:S62–S73.

Passias, Thanasis. 1996. Effects of hypoglycemia on thermoregulatory responses. *Journal of Applied Physiology* 80(3):1021–1032.

Schroeder, Jan. 1997. A comparison of three fluid replacement strategies for maintaining euhydration during prolonged exercise. *Canadian Journal of Applied Physiology* 22(1):48–57.

Terrados, N. 1995. Exercise in the heat: Strategies to minimize the adverse effects on performance. *Journal of Sports Sciences* 13:S55–S62.

Tochihara, Yutaka. 1995. Effects of repeated cold exposures to severely cold environments on thermal responses to humans. *Ergonomics* 38(5):987–995.

Wexler, Randall. 2002. Evaluation and treatment of heat-related illness. *American Family Physician* 65(11):2307–2314.

Learning Skills

Ahern, David. 1997. Psychosocial factors in sports injury rehabilitation. *Clinics in Sports Medicine* 16(4):755–764.

Bortoli, Laura. 1992. Effect of contextual interference on learning technical sports skills. *Perceptual and Motor Skills* 75:555–562.

Cox, Richard. *Sports Psychology: Concepts and Applications.* Fourth Edition. Burr Ridge, IL: WCB/McGraw-Hill, 1998.

Havari, H. 1996. Effects of mental practice on performance are moderated by cognitive anxiety as measured by the Sport Competition Anxiety Test. *Perceptual and Motor Skills* 83:1375–1383.

Kohl, Robert. 1992. Alternating actual and imagery practice: Preliminary theoretical considerations. *Research Quarterly for Exercise and Sport* 63(2):162–170.

Lee, Timothy. 1991. What is repeated in a repetition? Effects of practice conditions on motor skill acquisition. *Physical Therapy* 71(2):150–156.

Magill, Richard. *Motor Learning: Concepts and Applications*. Fifth Edition. Burr Ridge, IL: WCB/McGraw-Hill, 1998.

McCullagh, Penny. 1997. Learning versus correct models: Influence of model type on the learning of a free weight squat lift. *Research Quarterly for Exercise and Sport* 68(1):56–61.

Schmidt, RA. 1975. A schema theory of discrete motor learning skills. *Psychology Review* 82: 225–260.

Schmidt, RA. 2003. Motor schema theory after 27 years: reflections and implications for a new theory. *Research Quarterly for Exercise and Sport* 74(4):366–375.

Shea, Charles. 1990. Specificity and variability of practice. *Research Quarterly for Exercise and Sport* 61(2):169–177. Stephan, K. M. 1996. Motor imagery: Anatomical representation and electrophysiological characteristics. *Neurochemical Research* 21:1105–1116.

Weeks, D. L. 1998. Relative frequency of knowledge of performance and motor skills learning. *Research Quarterly for Exercise and Sport* 69(3):224–230.

White, Allison. 1996. Use of different imagery perspectives on the learning and performance of different motor skills. *The British Journal of Psychology* 86:169–180.

Wrisberg, Craig. 1991. The effect of contextual variety on the practice, retention, and transfer of an applied motor skill. *Research Quarterly for Exercise and Sport* 62(4):406–412.

Performance and Injuries

Barry, Nicole. 1996. Overuse syndrome in adult athletes. *Rheumatic Diseases Clinics of North America* 22(3):515–530.

Benhaddad, Aissa. 1999. Early hemorheologic aspects of overtraining in elite athletes. *Clinical Hemorheology and Microcirculation* 20:117–125.

Best, Thomas. 1997. Soft tissue injuries and muscle tears. *Clinics in Sports Medicine* 16(3):419–434.

Budgett, Richard. 1998. Fatigue and underperformance in athletes: The overtraining syndrome. *The British Journal of Sports Medicine* 32:107–110.

Cantu, Robert. 1998. Return to play guidelines after a head injury. *Clinics in Sports Medicine* 17(1):46–59.

Cross, Kevin M. 2003. Training and equipment to prevent athletic head and neck injuries. *Clinics in Sports Medicine* 22(3):639–667

Derman, W. 1997. The "worn out athlete": A clinical approach to chronic fatigue in athletes. *Journal of Sports Sciences* 15:341–351.

Fry, Andrew. 1997. Resistance exercise overtraining and overreaching: Neuroendocrine responses. *Sports Medicine* 23(2):106–129.

Garrett, William. 1996. Muscle strain injuries. *American Journal of Sports Medicine* 24(6):PS0002–PS0008.

Gibalas, M. J. 1994. The effects of tapering on strength performance in trained athletes. *International Journal of Sports Medicine* 15:492–497.

Grandjean, Ann. 1999. Nutritional requirements to increase lean body mass. *Clinics in Sports Medicine* 18(3):623–632.

Handbook of Adolescent Medicine. *Adolescent Medicine,* Volume 14, Number 2, June 2003, 183–524.

Ireland, Mary Lloyd. 2004. Special concerns of female athletes. *Clinics in Sports Medicine* 23(2):281–298.

Kenetta, Goran. 1998. Overtraining and recovery: A conceptual model. *Sports Medicine* 26(1):1–16.

Knapp, Thomas. 1997. Stress fractures: General concepts. *Clinics in Sports Medicine* 16(2):339–356.

Lehmann, M. J. 1997. Training and overtraining: An overview and experimental results in endurance sports. *Journal of Sports Medicine and Physical Fitness* 37:7–17.

Mackinnon, L. T. 1997. Immunity in athletes. *International Journal of Sports Medicine* 18:(Supplement 1):S62–S68.

Manore, Melinda. 1999. Nutritional needs of the female athlete. *Clinics in Sports Medicine* 18(3):549–563.

McHugh, Malachy. 1999. The role of passive muscle stiffness in symptoms of exercise-induced muscle damage. *American Journal of Sports Medicine* 27(5):594–599.

Morton, R. H. 1997. Modeling training and overtraining. *Journal of Sports Sciences* 15:335–340.

Mujika, I. 1998. The influence of training characteristics and tapering on the adaptation in highly trained individuals: A review. *International Journal of Sports Medicine* 19:439–446.

Peter, John. 1998. Infectious mononucleosis. *Pediatrics in Review* 19(8):276–279.

Plutonian, Margot. 1998. The female athletic triad. *Clinics in Sports Medicine* 17(4):675–693.

Saperstein, Alan. 1996. Pediatric and adolescent sports medicine. *Pediatric Clinics of North America* 43(5):P1013–P1033.

Snyder, A. C. 1993. A physiological/psychological indicator of overreaching during intensive training. *International Journal of Sports Medicine* 14:29–32.

Treiber, Frank et al. 1998. Effects of theraband and lightweight dumbbell training on shoulder rotation torque and serve performance in college tennis players. *American Journal of Sports Medicine* 26(4):510–515.

Urhausen, Alex. 1995. Blood hormones as markers of training stress and over-training. *Sports Medicine* 20(4):251–276.

Wilder, Robert P. January 2004. Overuse injuries: Tendinopathies, stress fractures, compartment syndrome, and shin splints. *Clinics in Sports Medicine* 23(1):55–81.

Wojtys, Edward. 1996. Neuromuscular adaptations in isokinetic, isotonic, and agility training programs. *American Journal of Sports Medicine* 24(2):187–192.

Zarkadas, P. C., 1995. Modelling the effects of taper on performance, maximal oxygen uptake, and the anaerobic threshold in endurance triathletes. *Modeling and Control of Ventilation.* Plenum Press, New York, 1995, 179–186.

978-0-595-36435-0
0-595-36435-7

Printed in the United States
55554LVS00003B/307-399

9 780595 364350